The Healing Blade

A
Tale
of
Neurosurgery

EDWARD J. SYLVESTER

Beck Press, Inc.
3404 S. McClintock Drive, Suite 859
Tempe, Arizona   85282
WWW: beckpress.amug.com

Designed by Michael Hagelberg

Manufactured in the United States of America

Beck Press Edition printed by

McNaughton & Gunn, Inc.

ISBN: 0-9660972-0-3

To Daniel and Katie with love

Acknowledgments

MOST OF THOSE who played key roles in this book appear as figures in the story. However, many others without whose help the book could not have been completed are not named inside.

Many neurosurgery department chairmen were generous with their time in giving me a picture of neurosurgery and the training of its practitioners in the United States, yet they are quoted at most only briefly in the manuscript. I would like to thank Dr. Peter Black of Harvard, Peter Bent Brigham Hospital; Dr. Joseph Ransohoff of New York University, Bellevue Medical Center; Dr. William Shucart of Tufts, New England Medical Center; Dr. Dennis Spencer of Yale, the Yale Medical Center; Dr. Bennett Stein of Columbia, the Neurological Institute; Dr. Charles Wilson of the University of California at San Francisco; and Dr. Nicholas Zervas of Harvard, Massachusetts General Hospital. In addition, dozens of neurosurgeons and residents at numerous medical centers aided me in understanding their specialty and its demands and rewards; I hope their efforts are reflected in the final product.

I would especially like to thank those whose duties make them part of the special entity called Barrow Neurological Institute, either now or during production of the first edition of *The Healing Blade*: Paula Ohlwiler, Hersh Garrett, Barbara Hecht, and the rest of the staff of Barrow Neurosurgical Associates; Toby Jardine and medical illustrator Mark Shornak of Barrow Neurological Institute; and Debbra Gelbart and Robin Cook of St. Joseph's Hospital.

Susan Fuchs of the Arizona Medical Association provided invaluable background information and assistance during my first years at work on the book.

Special thanks to Cynthia Knapp, a fellow science writer, for her recollection of *The Great Soul Trial* by John Grant Fuller, with its insight into events of the early days of Barrow Neurological Insitute.

My recounting of the early days of the Phoenix area comes from a variety of sources culled over twenty-five years, but at several key points I relied on the writings of Marshall Trimble, one of Arizona's renowned story-tellers.

And finally, my deepest thanks to my editors, past and present: Marilyn Abraham, who edited the hard-cover edition while a vice president of Simon & Schuster, and Conrad Storad of Beck Press. The cover and typography of the Beck Press Edition are the work of graphic artist Michael Hagelberg, whose illustrations and designs have won dozens of major, national awards.

CONTENT

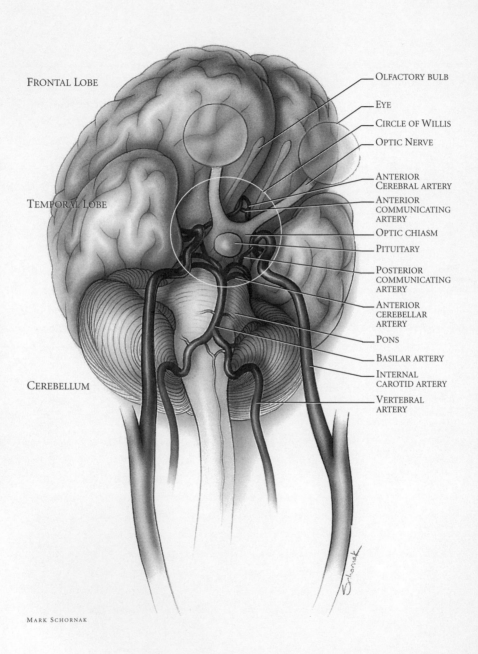

FRONTAL LOBE

TEMPORAL LOBE

CEREBELLUM

OLFACTORY BULB

EYE

CIRCLE OF WILLIS

OPTIC NERVE

ANTERIOR
CEREBRAL ARTERY

ANTERIOR
COMMUNICATING
ARTERY

OPTIC CHIASM

PITUITARY

POSTERIOR
COMMUNICATING
ARTERY

ANTERIOR
CEREBELLAR
ARTERY

PONS

BASILAR ARTERY

INTERNAL
CAROTID ARTERY

VERTEBRAL
ARTERY

MARK SCHORNAK

THE DRAMATIC FOCUS OF *THE HEALING BLADE* is a procedure called the standstill, developed for neurosurgery about ten years ago. For a patient, what is "standing still"—at zero on every meter—is each measure of life known to medical science. A person undergoing a standstill has no breath, no heartbeat, no blood flow, no viable temperature, and most important, no brainwaves or other brain activity that clinically define being alive.

The standstill is fascinating in its implications at a time when theologians, cosmologists and many of the rest of us wonder aloud if something human survives death and if there is an individual spirit that can transcend time and place and molecular substance, since whether something actually does so or not appears beyond resolution. The standstill does not answer the question, but it offers a fascinating place to look. Patients are taken down to death itself and brought back again. That much is certain.

These stories take place at Barrow Neurological Institute in Phoenix, Arizona, where more standstills have been done, and done with more successful outcomes, than anywhere else in the world. Initially I set out to write a book on the brain, wondering how such a vast topic might be narrowed. The neurosurgical operating room, the only place the living brain is actually exposed to eyes and touch, seemed a fascinating place to start. It was not long before the fight for life of real people emerged as the drama, the tale. Inevitably, looking over the shoulder and trying to see through the eyes of one of the world's great neurosurgeons at one of the major neurological institutes became the compelling twin focus. But to paraphrase T.S. Eliot, In our end is our beginning, in our beginning our end. For me, and I hope for readers, the world first glimpsed in "The Power of Resolution" ultimately opens out into the mysterious universe of the brain itself.

These are all true stories; the writer is a reporter, no more or less. No quotes have been altered or imagined, no names have been changed, and no endings have been given a happy spin or edited out. There are no compound characters, and scenes that may appear imagined are all rendered through the eyes of one or more witnesses, but most often I am the witness. I did not pick operations to write about, in the style of some popular magazines, in which the ending had already turned out happily as I began writing, leaving the drama "cooked" from the outset and the reader manipulated. However, like every journalist, I am responsible for focusing on some stories more than others, and for skill or lack of it in telling them. I witnessed their unfolding, usually the whole of it, but more importantly they grabbed and held me. There are no pseudonyms in *The Healing Blade*. If unable to reach a patient for permission, I used only his or her first name and last initial; no patients refused to be identified.

Every story has one overarching point of view, that of the story-teller. I am responsible for any misstatements, distortions of perspective, or omissions of fact, though I made my very best effort to avoid all of those. Perhaps most important of all to a work of journalism, none of the major subjects of this book read it in advance, nor did anyone at Barrow Neurological Institute approve any part of its contents. The sole exception to this is the narrative of the Morbidity and Mortality Conference beginning on page 138. No one attending these "M&Ms" is allowed to take any form of notes or to take any paper handed out for discussion, nor can the discussions themselves be continued outside. Those prohibitions apply to everyone, including the BNI director. No one outside BNI may even sit in on M&M conferences. To my knowledge, those rules are universal in American medical institutions. I was permitted to attend any M&M conference I chose without advance notice, to take notes, and to carry the notes out with me. In return for that unique privilege, I agreed that any passage of the book reporting on an M&M conference would be approved by Dr. Robert F. Spetzler, in order to protect the confidentiality of the patients and physicians involved. Although this was not part of the bargain, I destroyed all M&M notes once I had used them.

The Healing Blade opens on Tuesday, April 25, 1989, and ends eight years later on Wednesday, August 20, 1997. The book originally was published in hardcover by Simon & Schuster in 1993, so the new edition represents a continued unfolding of a story that will never come to a conclusion. This offered a unique challenge in attempting to prepare this edition. "New edition" implies that the author has gone back and altered much of the original text to improve its currency and perspective. That was precisely what I could not do, because I did not want to offer a revisionist view of the past. As a result, to preserve the integrity of the earlier stories, the only changes I made to the original material were in correcting bona fide errors, of which there were mercifully few, thanks to expert medical readers and terrific editors at Simon & Schuster.

The forecasts made in 1992 as the hardcover went to press are seen by the conclusion of the Beck Press edition with the advantage of five years' perspective. They remain remarkably current, thanks to the vision of the sources. Thus, although a substantial amount of the text has been changed or added, it is all at the end of the book. Chapter Nine opens just as the hardcover version did, but now there is a transition midway through as the story moves beyond its original ending toward the present. Chapter Ten is entirely new and has never appeared before.

A good, true story is like river rafting—wild but not too wild, controlled but not too much so. The stories themselves rather than the writer's imagination offer the powerful and different currents pulling onward, sometimes breathtakingly fast, sometimes very gently. There are eddies that slow, where you can get pulled in and feel becalmed. If at times the natural excitement of these stories bogs down in explanation, I apologize. I simplified the best I could for the general reader, trying to compromise when necessary between the precise view of the physician and a clear view for the reader. The more you want to know, the more you can let yourself be drawn into the more challenging passages. However, if you really want only the powerful currents, let them pull you. The stories won't be lost if you pass by the more technical passages, but they won't drag you down if you stay with them awhile. For me, *The Healing Blade's* fictional kin is the techno-thriller and it can be read in the same ways.

Far more importantly, there are emotional upheavals here beyond my control or anyone else's, and the reader should know that going in.

People die, sometimes with all the world pulling for them; others survive utterly unbelievable odds to live, sometimes when hardly anyone seems to care. Even Dr. Robert Spetzler, one of the world's great neurosurgeons by the judgment of his peers, has very limited control over the outcomes of his efforts. That's the point, finally. In the neurosurgeon's perfect world, the dangers, however terrifying, all would end in good outcomes, wrought by flawless skill and judgment. There would be no ugly surprises, and everyone would go home as good as new. These stories are of the world we actually live in. Here's to that other world and those who try to make it so.

ED SYLVESTER
TEMPE, ARIZONA
SEPTEMBER 1997

The Power of Resolution

IN THE BEGINNING, the brain was singular, whole and undivided. That was the problem. Like the Earth of Genesis, the brain as an object of knowledge, and so of treatment and healing, was without form, its secrets hidden in a fog from which it seemed clarity would never emerge. The brain needed discrimination into all its structures and colorings, the enumerated chambers and scaffolds; it needed articulation that could account for the splendors of the universe it created within itself. It needed resolving into the millions of complex and subtle actions, apprehensions, sallies, dances and chants with which it could engage its universe.

Just over a century ago, the brain was like an image under a microscope that is beyond the instrument's power of resolution, a spheroid blob that might really be one object of entirely different shape than appears, or a number of objects all of different shapes. No way of telling.

When you twist up the magnification of a microscope that is already beyond its power to resolve, in place of a tiny spheroid blob you see a large spheroid blob. It doesn't matter how much the image is magnified; at Earth-size, an Earth-size blob comes up. It only improves if you also increase the resolution of the microscope.

Overwhelming though it had seemed, the quest to understand the brain at submicroscopic resolution succeeded, magnificently. By now, the time of this story, a century's unrelenting effort to articulate the brain into its tiniest anatomical structures and most detailed physiological activities was in its final stages, a century that had seen the invention of the most dazzling technology in history and the bending of much of that technology to this purpose.

But as great an adventure is now under way, and that is what this story is about. A revolution is going on in neurosurgery and neurology that those in its midst believe will make the era before this seem like a dark age—like Europe as the cathedrals emerged with the millennium, as both evidence of monumental change coming and framework of that change. As then, the forms, designs and crafts that produced those stone works of highest art had existed before, on that same soil in ancient times, on Eastern soil at that time. But a new design had taken root.

The cathedrals that emerged were a product of their time and place and the minds of the men and women whose spirit they embodied, and of the force of their will directed in new ways, as though the spirit of the new millennium were to be felt in shaping space before it had any content.

This is as much a story of our time and place. Over a three-year period I spent hundreds of days and nights at Barrow Neurological Institute, in downtown Phoenix. The institute is part of St. Joseph's Hospital and Medical Center and to the unsuspecting eye is indistinct from it. You have to be told that the halls of Barrow are polished dark stone, while those of St. Joe's are carpeted, to realize you have made a transition. But sure as the cathedrals marked an unmistakable reach for heaven, there at Barrow is a giant structure within which everything and everyone focuses inward to the brain, from the neurosurgical suites on the fourth floor to the autopsy rooms and laboratories in the basement, to the giant toruses of CT and MRI scanners, intraoperative microscopes, three-dimensional television sets to view surgeries, all to bring the brain into focus.

A large part of the story involves the amassing of ever-more sophisticated technology, ever-more dazzling machinery to see the brain in dozens of different ways, to measure its every input and output and response to every imaginable drug.

But what has that technology brought us? The answers to that question are not unequivocal ones. This is a story of disasters as well as triumphs, and of stars to be sure—some of them on the receiving end of the knife.

The story is shaped by overarching, powerful personalities. They shaped Barrow Neurological Institute; they shaped neurosurgery. You don't do that from the sidelines and you don't get to the center of the action by waiting to be called. You know and go. What goes on inside brain surgeons' brains? What makes them go? Monumental ego? Or, in the words of Peter Raudzens, chief of neuroanesthesia, big brass balls? To crack open a living human's skull and put a razor to his brain. Make that his soul. What kind of people do this sort of thing for a living?

Robert Spetzler, director of BNI, is a man of supreme and unshakeable confidence. Spetzler is tall, with a handsome face, reddish brown hair, and mustache. A contrast with white-haired John Green, who created Barrow out of cowtown dust and who introduced us in Green's office. In the elderly Green, a man of kindness and good humor, it is hard to see the virile medical giant. Spetzler remembers him that way.

Spetzler still has the rangy, powerful build of the varsity backstroker he was twenty years ago. Then swimmers were first being taught to push into the wall of pain as they overextend muscles and oxygen demand, to push until they broke through the pain barrier into a pure concentration of will on swimming. Appropriate for the neurosurgeon.

As medical legend has it, the cardiovascular and orthopedic surgeons are the power athletes; it takes a lot of physical strength to crack a chest and rearrange bones. But the pure concentration, hour after hour, the force of will that can carry an operating team from morning until night and then, in just the moment of repose, jump back into a sheer emergency at full mental force, that is the brain surgeon's forte, physical power held together by strength of will as much as muscular coordination.

At the climax of this story, a moment as self-defined and unequivocal as its beginning, Spetzler and I were talking in Vienna, Austria, on an off day in the middle of what was already proving to be the most difficult surgery he had ever been through. We were talking about what a neurosurgeon does to prepare for a major case like this. "You go over the procedure, and over it again, and over it again," he said. "You simply repeat every step you are going to do and go through every possible thing that can go wrong. And then you do it again."

You go over the procedure so often that it cannot leave your mind; that's the point. Then it is the night before surgery. "As you drift down to sleep, you are in the operating room, and you cut the wrong side. Or you see a vein or artery, and you cut right through it. Stupid things, all the things you prepared yourself never to do in your first day of residency, you're doing them. And that wakes you up. And then you think about the procedure, and as you fall asleep, it comes again. On the night before a major case, of course, you never really sleep. You half-sleep. Running things through your mind."

And then after a repose full of nightmares, you go in and do the procedure, calm and cool, truly the most confident human alive. Procedure is the key word to neurosurgery. A procedure has specified steps that can and must be choreographed and rehearsed; it has a beginning, a middle and an end. Most importantly, it must not have surprises.

Well and good, but where do I begin. For weeks I fumbled through stacks of notes, boxes of tapes, the bones of history, for omens, like some ancient hunter trying to guess where the game lies, but came up only with the same annoying, finally angering metaphor—a gray blob, as large as you choose it to be but a frustrating, enraging, indiscriminate blob no matter how large you magnify it, however powerful your vision. Then, as sometimes happens, the point came, and it came in precisely this way.

On April 16, I jolted awake for no reason at 4:20 a.m. and within a few minutes was running off the shivers in the dark, by far the earliest I've been out running in ten years. I started my stopwatch as always and heard the mounting roar of a motorcycle headed south, fast, beyond the wall ahead as I ran east, where the sky was still pitch dark. Then there was a scraping clash of cheap metal, like a hubcap clattering off. I figured it was just that and ran on as the motorcycle roared southward.

Seconds later someone shouted, yelling like an angry brawler; then came an undertone of pain. I turned out to the main road. In the dark I could just make out someone writhing, sitting up, lying down, shadow on shadow, then shouting again. He lay in the dirt of the broad shoulder, out of further danger. Farther down the road, illuminated by a street-light, the motorcycle lay on its side. I had nearly reached him, out-shouting him to lie still, when I picked out something much more alarming than his pain. Stretched across the fast lane, face down and arms outstretched and pointed like a diver's, lay a second figure in clothing as dark as the road.

Running to the dark, blurry form I heard the easy breathing of someone deeply asleep, and stood in front of him facing the lights curving toward us in the dark, waving my arms. The pickup truck swerved and stopped. *Call 911!* He nodded and drove on. Now the breathing was of a troubled dreamer, halting, beginning again, only now with a sucking sound I had gotten to know over the past three years, following neurosurgery residents into the Emergency Room when such accident cases were brought in. I couldn't make out his face; it was topped by unruly brown hair. No helmet. I thought, He's dying and needs CPR, but I knew better than to try to move him with a likely neck injury. A mixture of dread and relief there. A man was dying at my feet, but there really wasn't anything I could do but dance like a rodeo clown to keep the trucks off him.

The next pickup was luck, a railroader with flares we set out. And the next a charm, an emergency med tech on his way to work. The sucking was more pronounced now. Another motorist was kneeling by the second boy, twenty yards away off the side of the road. Here, the railroader and I slowly rolled the body while the paramedic turned the head in precise unison. A very young face appeared, not 20 yet and, I thought, maybe as old as he gets. Placing a plastic shield over the boy's mouth, routine in the era of AIDS, the paramedic began mouth-to-mouth. The sucking sound went on. Somewhere inside the seemingly undamaged skull I guessed blood was leaking, probably throttling the brain stem, where breathing and heartbeat are regulated, the animal soul.

Cops were here now. The boy jolted and clear fluid poured out of his mouth, drained down the roadbed. The EMT stopped and pumped hard on the boy's chest, three times, went back to the mouth-to-mouth. Was he dying? More police cars, finally ambulances. The boy was put on a respirator, his breathing steady and regular; now his heartbeat would sound fine, I knew. Statements for the police report: "He coded almost right away," the EMT said; not much older than the boy and looking the most upset of anyone.

Sure, he was the only one who had a prayer of saving him, so the only one who can wonder if everything will turn out all right and if he did everything right. It looked right.

I thought the other boy probably wasn't hurt too bad, as aware of his pain and circumstances as he was, asking over and over how his friend was doing. He was hurt just bad enough to blurt it all.

Two pals drinking it up, roaring off into the night. Sucking down whiskey and springtime and life. Hit the guardrail at sixty and both got thrown off the bike, which roared on riderless for nearly a hundred yards before skidding off the road. That eerie image won't go away, the riderless motorcycle roaring south, something I heard but never saw. Now I see it all the time but hear nothing, a little silent movie in my head. It was the driver at my feet, and, as it would occur to any spectator, it occurred to me. What will happen at the other end of the ambulance ride? Recovery? I doubted it. Dead on arrival? Yes and no, and the point turns on this. The respirator would mimic life to a T. Death would be a matter of decision. What had once been unequivocal and immediate would be debated over time. Was that all we had won with the glitzy chrome technology?

The newspaper said that the boy was eighteen and that he died later that April day in the hospital; so be it. Was death at 4:40, 4:50, or when the respirator was turned off? Had his parents had the finances or lacked the will, death might have been stamped days or weeks or months later. In the interim the staff on dawn rounds would have written, as I'd seen the neurosurgery residents write dozens of times, *Patient remains in a vegetative state. Glasgow Coma Scale of 3. Does not respond to commands, does not respond to touch, pupils non-responsive and fully dilated, does not respond to pain....*

I did not witness the hours between the accident and the pronouncement of death this time, but I had many times before. The incidents all have one quality in common, and one in particular now stood in sharp relief— an accident of over a year earlier that had faded from memory came back crystal clear.

Paul Francis, then a first-year neurosurgical resident, and I were having lunch in the cafeteria when the trauma bells rang. We rushed to the trauma room and waited. As Hollywood suspense is built by music, the tension in the ER is driven by the sound of sirens, faint then distinct, rising to crescendo, then stopping; that's when you hold your breath. Then you hear the rumble of wheels and the rapid pumping of feet shoving the gurney like a battering ram first through the electric doors into the ER and then through the rubber curtain into the trauma room. I ducked out of the way as the trauma team rushed to hook up IVs, respirator, monitors, to take pulse, insert catheter, knowing Paul would call out if something instructive occurred once the patient was stabilized.

It always took a while before the rush of green scrubs cleared and revealed the patient. This one was a motorcycle crash on one of Arizona's desert highways. A young man in his 20s, handsome as the devil with curly light brown hair and a reddish mustache, slumbering but otherwise appearing just fine. His breathing was regular and even, though you couldn't tell if it was his own or only the respirator's; his heart beat steady and true.

"No helmet?" Paul Francis asked.

"He had a helmet," the paramedic said, pausing for effect, "hanging on his seat."

Francis looked into one gray eye, saw its pupil dilated wide and called to me. "His right pupil is blown, he's in bad shape. I don't know what's wrong. Everything else seems fine. And his left. Both pupils blown. What the hell is wrong." Francis pinched the man's nipple, which will bring a stir even from someone fairly comatose. Nothing.

One of the nurses, seeing a line of blood in the man's hair rubbed it back with her glove, a gentle gesture, and suddenly everyone, leaning in so intently, sucked in a breath. A palm-size piece of his skull lifted up right at his hairline; his brain surface was splattered underneath. And the nurse said in one of those clear hard voices that speak years of this, "We're looking right at his sinuses." And so we were. Right down through the roof of the world.

The trauma surgeon looked in at him and barked, "Turn off the respirator."

The chest fell still, eyes stared wide and vacant, and the heart monitor went off into that long inane peal when the beats no longer come, when the brain stem has ceased sending its pulses and the heart's own signals fibrillate. He had looked so lifelike.

Where has this technology brought us, other than to the brink of bankruptcy?

Sometimes it has brought us to a chronic vegetative state instead of a quick death. Sometimes all we get is a big gray blur where a moment of terror used to be.

There it is.

The line of death, razor sharp and sudden as a hammer blow, has been magnified and magnified and magnified yet again. The thin gray twilight line now can go on forever. Without resolution. And that, to be sure, is the darkness out of which this story emerges and into which its protagonists fight to prevent its sinking. New science often has a way of magnifying like that, boosting raw power by orders of magnitude without articulating it into useable pathways. It gives the power to see but does not give vision itself. It is not a gift outright.

The frustration of watching someone on a respirator for as long as the power is kept on is the same as the frustration when it seems the combined genius of the century has netted nuclear bombs. What is power without resolution? A great gray blob. How then do you bend the enormous powers of new science to your will? How do you articulate, discriminate, increase the resolution?

Focus, first. Concentrate every fiber at your command to this one thing. Neurosurgery is about winning resolution, in all the ways it can be won, for those are all the ways it can be lost; it is about harnessing technological power, bending it to one's hand by one's will. The story is about the articulation of consciousness, layer by painstaking layer, and that is the same as the articulation of death, layer by layer.

The razor line between life and death is crossed when you hit the rail at 60, no matter how you magnify the line. But the difference between that death and the "deaths" in standstill procedures in neurosurgery is the difference between hurling tons of metal into the ground and landing the space shuttle. There it is.

Articulate, discriminate, control, control more precisely. Focus to the maximum power of resolution, then focus on increasing the power of resolution. To win you must take each emergence of the gray blob as a challenge; you have reached the limit of your resolution, which must have no limit. On and on. Western science and medicine, it is argued, are about ever-increasing control over the unknown, over uncertainty and the unexpected. Neurosurgery is the paradigm, without apology.

You see what the gray blob is now, so tiny it is just beyond the limit of your straining eyes and it may be about to do something, now looming so large it fills the entirety of your vision and your mind with its grayness. No difference. It is the enemy.

Standstill

JACK SCHULTE is a stubborn but good-humored man, all 64 years of him. As a young marine, he'd fought—and joked—his way across the South Pacific, and the stubbornness and humor showed all the way. When the going got tough, on Guadalcanal, or Guam, or Okinawa, you fired off a few jokes and you got through. That was years ago, but the habits of life do not retire with you to Sun City, in the middle of the Arizona desert. Only April and the temperature was through the ceiling, in the nineties and not even noon yet. But there was the matter of the giant saguaro cactus that had taken a dive in Jack's front yard, and it was not going to stay there. Schulte took an ax to it, and right in the middle of a swing, *he* went down.

The world spun, his vision dimmed, doubled. His head was splitting. Two neighbors rushed to his side and as they helped him into the house, Schulte saw that his left foot was dragging. "My God, I've had a stroke," he said. Not quite, but almost. Deep within his brain, far too deep for any surgeon to reach under ordinary circumstances, a major artery had ballooned out, like a weakened inner tube about to rupture. When it blows, the soul blows with it. But for now, it hung there, an aneurysm puffed out, causing horrible pain but holding steady.

WEDNESDAY, APRIL 26

Tom Grahm left Operating Room 1 just before 8 a.m., his first neurosurgery of the day already behind him. The chief resident of Barrow Neurological Institute in Phoenix, he had completed an operation to cleanse an artery that had become clogged with plaque, this time on one of the two carotid arteries leading up the neck into the brain of a sixty-six-year-old woman.

Plaque contains little stony flakes. Even before it builds far enough to block the massive heart arteries, the powerful pressure of blood pumped straight upward can blow off a single flake from the carotid lining. That flake will head north into the brain, to course along ever-narrowing arterial branches until it hits a juncture too small for it to pass; there it will block all or part of the blood supply beyond it.

The left and right carotids are the major arteries leading from the heart to the head, and each splits into internal and external branches. The internal carotids, along the side of the neck, carry about half the brain's supply of blood. The other half comes from the vertebral arteries that follow the front of the spinal cord.

Of all the demands on the heart for blood, none is as critical or as complex as the brain's. One hundred billion cells constantly demand oxygen, the fuel of cellular metabolism—less when we sleep, more whenI we're brainstorming, but always without interruption. Interrupt the blood flow long enough and brain tissue dies; the common term for that death of brain tissue from lost oxygen is stroke.

Stroke was the major threat in the surgery Grahm had just performed, and in the landmark surgery that was to follow, but it was certainly a lot easier to understand in terms of the relatively routine procedure on which he had just assisted.

The vascular (as in vessel) system of the brain is a masterpiece of evolutionary engineering, a network that on film looks much like a tumbleweed: thick stalks of arteries at the base, branching at Y-junctures, branching again into ever-thinner offshoots that, constrained by the shape of the brain, curl into an overall hemisphere. Growing ever finer, the arteries supply oxygen to ever-smaller clusters of brain cells until finally, even under the intraoperative microscope, the tiny arteries called perforators seem mere root hairs against the giant trunks of major vessels.

Block off a blood vessel with plaque and you block all its tributaries. Then one of two things happens. The flake dissolves in the caustic and turbulent stream of blood, and in the mind's eye a cloud may seem to pass, a momentary darkening, and then all is well again. Or the flake might lodge longer— say, hours—though perhaps other blood vessels are helping to supply the region. Interruption of normal blood flow is called ischemia, and when blood stops flowing, it immediately begins to clot. In the throes of a transitory ischemic activity, or TIA, the mind's eye may dim, the beholder lapsing into semi-consciousness, losing bearings, slurring speech, yet have all those return bright as morning in hours or days if plaque and clot dissolve. If the interruption of blood flow does not clear, on its own or with medication, cells begin to die. Cerebral infarct—the medical term for stroke, death of brain tissue due to lost blood supply, a permanent darkening of some part of the beholder's universe that may be minor, major or total.

Grahm flopped down on the leather couch in the men's lounge off the surgical dressing room, not bothering to remove his scrub cap or glasses, his mask tugged down around his neck and the sleeves of his operating gown pulled around his hands, balled into the fetal position required to jam his lanky frame onto the couch. Inured to the constant din of the television permanently on in the lounge, Grahm dove toward the kind of snooze residents learn to survive on during six years of unremittingly intense training—though now in his final year, he and co-chief Fred Williams did not have to pace themselves through thirty-six and forty-eight hour sleepless shifts any longer.

Now his days might be long and nights short, but he got to spend them at home with his wife, instead of here on a cot. Still, he particularly wanted a nap today. The case following in OR 1 was the kind no resident could afford to miss, although it was Williams who would assist in surgery.

Robert Spetzler, Barrow's director, would attempt to clip off a giant basilar aneurysm—a ballooning of the basilar artery—at a site virtually inaccessible, deep in the brain of a sixty-four-year-old man named Jack Schulte. The surgery Grahm had just completed, delicate as it was, was the routine end of neurosurgery. What would follow was off the scale. Or better put: off just about everyone's scale but Spetzler's.

To get to the aneurysm, the surgical team would perform a hypothermic arrest. This procedure was being attempted in neurosurgery in few other hospitals anywhere in the world, yet because of Spetzler, Barrow had logged enough of them to publish a study of seven cases in the *Journal of Neurosurgery*. And in a period when nearly all such procedures were ending in death or severe neurological impairment, the BNI paper reported that out of its seven, four patients had had "excellent" outcomes; one had a "good" outcome, left with a slight nerve palsy; one was "fair," with partial paralysis on one side; and only one had died. The critical point was that all the patients would have died for certain without surgery, and there was no other way to do the surgery than by using this high-risk procedure.

The nickname for hypothermic arrest is "standstill," a properly stark metaphor. The patient would be put into a barbiturate coma, to radically cut his brain's use of oxygen. His blood then would be circulated through a bypass pump and his heart stopped, just as in heart bypass surgery. Then the blood would be chilled, pumped back into the body to refrigerate the brain far below room temperature.

Hypothermic arrest was developed by cardiac surgeons in the 1960s; the procedure made such heart surgery as transplants survivable. But the initial idea was to continue pumping blood to all organs except the heart while the heart was being operated on. The neurosurgeon's version of the procedure went to the limit. Schulte's heart would be stopped. But once the proper low brain temperature was reached, the blood would be drained from his body instead of continuing to circulate on a bypass pump.

Now, for a period of up to an hour, no blood and therefore no oxygen would reach any cell in the patient's brain or any other organ. *You know the technical term for that condition,* one of the neurosurgeons had quipped. *It's called death.* Indeed, Schulte would be, by any medical definition, dead.

Then they would bring him back, and that is not supposed to be possible. The layman's awe at such a notion was filling Operating Room 1 with observers: a writer, and an entire television news crew from Sacramento. The news crew had come merely to interview Spetzler and get "dry run" footage for a documentary on hypothermic arrest. The procedure was so rare that even here they had no realistic hope of getting to film one. They had had the good fortune to arrive today, the first day in nearly a year when a standstill would be performed at Barrow.

During that year, Barrow was the busiest neurosurgical service in America, which might be of little general interest, but to Grahm it spoke volumes. To residents, operations are the job experience that launches careers. Actually, if they aspire to the pinnacle of medicine, an academic position in a university-affiliated hospital, there are three critical categories on the curriculum vitae: operations, publications in refereed medical journals, and presentations at medical conferences.

Grahm already had six publications under his belt, had made eleven conference presentations and operated almost daily. Many chiefs would be happy to conclude residency with one or two refereed publications, and in some programs, especially in the malpractice-litigious East, residents got little operating experience until they were at the chief level.

Being on a busy service wasn't the only critical requirement for an ambitious young neurosurgeon—and all young neurosurgeons are ambitious. Equally important was having a hand in important cases, and that meant working under a chair of neurosurgery with a big enough reputation to bring in referrals from across the country, someone to whom a neurologist in New York or California or Arkansas might refer a particularly tough and rare case. Spetzler was just that neurosurgeon, the cases he drew the most challenging, frequently deemed impossible by others; and the standstill the perfect showcase for his talents.

Grahm dove for his nap, but he never got close. His pager went off with its steam-whistle sound, and the number that followed was for the trauma room downstairs in emergency. He called, then took off like a shot. He managed to get back just in time to see the boss begin the standstill, not yet knowing that in the half hour he was in the trauma room he had already taken part in events that would put Spetzler and Barrow on network television and in the magazines of the world. More than that. How to describe the odds on what was unfolding? You watch a coin tossed, and it lands on its edge, a rare enough event to bring an *ahh* or two. Now the second toss lands on edge, bringing silence. And what do you say on the third? Here was the first toss of the coin.

IN OR 1, THE PATIENT is so thoroughly draped in green that only his brain shows, so it seems disembodied and curiously unreal, too *at hand* to be locus of all we identify as the human signature.

Three pounds of flesh, give or take; the most specialized set of 100 billion neurons known in the universe, and the most delicate, as complex as any planet, the product of a billion years of evolution; three pounds of flesh all the same.

Jack was always a guy to tackle things head on, Shirley Schulte had said, and after forty years of marriage there must have been a lot of "head ons" encompassed in her gentle smile.

After his spell in the morning, they went to the local hospital, but nothing showed on the x-ray or CT scan. For more than a day, Schulte fought a splitting headache with Tylenol and couldn't keep food down.

"Let me tell you how Jack is," Shirley had said. "Once he was working on his table top saw and sliced the tip of his thumb off. He drove himself to the Emergency Room. They stitched it up. He drove himself home, knocked back a shot of bourbon, and went to bed. No painkillers, no complaints. That's Jack."

Finally, Jack was air-evaced to St. Joe's yesterday when his doctor spotted a shadow on a scan that made him think of an aneurysm deep down under the brain's massive cerebrum, near where the higher brain emerges from the primitive brain stem. The vertebral arteries arise near the aorta and follow the front of the spinal cord into the brain stem. Part way up the brain stem the left and right vertebrals do something unusual for blood vessels. Instead of branching into finer tubes, they combine into the single, massive basilar artery. The basilar artery quickly begins sending offshoots to supply the higher brain stem and cerebellum with blood. Nowhere else in the brain do so many major arteries join and split, so this region is especially vulnerable to aneurysm. Nowhere else is the brain so inaccessible. Schulte's lesion was all but inoperable.

"In World War II, Jack's older brother, whom he adored, got drafted," Shirley said. "Jack couldn't bear that so he made his folks sign permission for him to enlist in the Marines at seventeen. His brother never went overseas. Jack was at Guadalcanal, Guam, Okinawa. And his buddies always said, just at the point they thought they were done for, Jack would think of something funny in the situation, and that got them through. That's Jack."

Where is Jack? Somewhere within these hemispheres and their blossoming stem, or in the totality, but here. Mood such as light-heartedness, sensations of pain, deeper sensations of emotional pain and joy. And traits much harder to put a finger on: a great sense of humor. A strong will. Deep love. We are conscious; not merely alive but aware of our lives; at magical times, supremely aware.

Damage the three pounds of tissue within the skull and much of what we identify as a person may be altered, maybe forever. Alter the flow of the blood or the particles it carries, or the flow of electric waves through the brain and you alter the human expression: beholder and beheld changed or vanished in a single moment.

How much is such a brain worth? That's neither an idle nor a cynical question. Value is being put on this brain right now, and that value has been growing exponentially for years. This is Godawful expensive: all the experiments, the training, the basic biology, animal studies, clinical trials, deaths on the table, deaths in the ward. And the worse-than-deaths, the "chronic vegetative states," so lifelike in intensive care; alive but not there. Behold: *nada*. How expensive it is to bring the man back depends on how hard it is. This is going to be hard.

The doctors who go into neurosurgery, unsurprisingly, take great pleasure in doing hard things, but sometimes they push that past where you think they can go.

Enter Spetzler, quietly. You know this is his OR today because Mozart is on the box. Joe Zabramski, Spetzler's protégé, always plays rock, which the Boss cannot bear. Spetzler is tall, six feet one inch, and still has the physique of the competitive swimmer. His brown hair and mustache have no hint of gray at forty-four, and a patient's wife once described him as "handsome as a movie star." Born in Germany but in the United States since he was nine years old, the son of an inventor credited as the "father of quartz clock." Well and good, but what makes *him* tick? Rather, what makes all of them tick, these brain surgeons routinely described by other high-powered doctors as believing they are more than human, that there is nothing they can't do?

First, they are trained, more carefully and more thoroughly and more rigidly than any Marine, to think they can do anything: to concentrate absolutely, to forget what limits of endurance are, to never falter or show doubt, to rehearse their routines more meticulously and thoroughly than anyone in any high-performing art. Being trained day and night, some have said, to believe they are gods and then prove it.

And the young ones, of course, seek out the masters. So the young backstroker from Illinois who broke and trained horses for a hobby went to Northwestern Medical School because the best neurosurgeon ran the progam there. When Paul Bucy retired before he could train Robert Spetzler, his mentor sent him to the University of California at San Francisco, because Bucy deemed Charles Wilson the best.

Spetzler recalls Wilson as "the most intense, concentrated bundle of energy on earth. He is wiry and lean and totally concentrated, not an ounce of fat on him. There is not an ounce of fat *in* him, or in his program. He has little patience with error and none for lack of dedication. He runs, sometimes fifteen miles, then performs neurosurgery. He is the most dedicated human I have ever seen, almost monklike in his devotion to neurosurgery, at the expense of a personal life, everything."

Ask neurosurgery heads around the country who's got the best neurosurgery residency now, nearly 20 years later, and Charlie Wilson is among three or four constantly named.

So Spetzler has one overriding ambition: to beat out his mentor and friend for that highest accolade. He doesn't say he wants to make Barrow's residency better than UCSF's. He just says he wants to make it the best in the country, and tells how his strategy differs from Wilson's.

Ask Charlie Wilson about his former chief resident:

"Cocky and self-assured to the point of arrogance," Wilson says without pause. "I have rarely seen anyone so confident in his abilities. But what terrific abilities."

Concentration, dedication. Spetzler alludes to these qualities often, sometimes indirectly. Asked what the most important skill is for a neurosurgeon, Spetzler says it is the ability to see , to project in three dimensions from seeing two-dimensional scans. But he is talking less about inborn vision than the result of studying the scans, and restudying them, and studying more. Studying them so intently before a big case that the night before you do not sleep, you play out the case, over and over, drifting into a half-sleep of nightmares.

The nightmares all arise from the same dark source. There is one word that is terror to every neurosurgeon, an innocent, even welcome word to most of us: surprise. Surprise can only mean that despite all your training and all your careful rehearsal of this procedure, something has gone dreadfully wrong, and now what do you do?

Where others see arrogance, Spetzler sees confidence, born of total focus and complete concentration. "The neurosurgeon must be completely confident in himself, in his skill. If he shows doubt or hesitation, even for a moment, that affects his entire team. And remember, this is a team effort, in which the entire team must work together with perfect precision. And sometimes maybe that confidence is mistaken for arrogance."

Maybe so. In a field in which stories on the grapevine routinely tell of neurosurgeons exploding in rage, screaming at underlings, some even hurling instruments, Spetzler rarely raises his voice.

No one ever reported hearing a tone of total frustration enter the smooth baritone. Not yet anyway. That would come much later, thousands of miles away.

THIS MIGHT BE MISSION CONTROL for a journey to another planet. Crowded into OR 1 are a television crew, staff, nurses; a mob. Large color television monitors peer down from the upper walls and offer the second-best view in the room, televising the brain as seen through the intraoperative microscope. The view is far better than over Spetzler's shoulder, because, magnified, the terrain takes on scope and grandeur appropriate to its importance; but it still lacks the depth you see directly through the binocular microscope, and that is a major loss.

Watch the lander descend, to a planet that is a human brain, that had been obscured by a cloud of bone now cleared away in the buzzing of the Midas Rex. The big, brass-headed bone saw looks as delicate as the pneumatic wrench in a gas station, fed by an equally prosaic green hose attached to compressed-air tanks in the corner, but it is part of the high-technology end of this supremely high-tech procedure. The Midas Rex, Spetzler says, is far more powerful than any other such tool, so you minimize the dangers of splintering bone, and thus of lodging deadly shards in the brain.

The intraoperative microscope itself is probably the major innovation that revolutionized neurosurgery, beginning about twenty-five years ago. With it, here among the indescribably delicate structures of the brain, if you were steady enough and focused enough, you could perform microneurosurgery. And then quickly, of course, few would perform any other kind of neurosurgery on a tough case. It is a stereo microscope, so the surgeon sees his work in three dimensions, the operating field looming large enough that filamentous nerves become thick white hoses. And equally important, of course, invisible structures are just barely perceived as filaments. The latest version of this microscope offers a zoom lens ranging from about five times magnification to about thirty-five times.

The microscope is operated by a lever held in Spetzler's mouth. leaving both hands free. His elbows rest on the arms of what looks like—and is called—a dentist's chair. The chair's height and horizontal motion are controlled with foot pedals, as is the Midas Rex saw. This technology, like the rest of the devices amid the tangle of wires in the operating room, tends to become invisible as time goes on, to recede into the background as the brain looms on the color monitor. The observer takes it for granted.

The operating room is crowded with a record twenty-four people, by the EEG tech's account, for there are two entirely separate surgical teams required, though they must work as harmoniously as any athletic team. "North," at the patient's head, are the neurosurgeons; "south," the cardiovascular surgeons; their domains cut in two by a blue curtain hung between them so surgeons of one group are not confused by orders given among the others. And the realm is split again: to the east, the heart-pump technicians with the giant chrome machine that will pump, oxygenate, and chill the blood to bring the patient's temperature down; to the west, the neuroanesthesiologists before a true mission-control array of monitors, each with an army of sine waves marching across its glowing green screen.

You must be careful in moving about. The first thing you learn is never to get near blue toweling, the signature of a sterile field. Everyone wears blue scrubs—green in some hospitals—with hair covering, masks and booties to match. But only those few who are scrubbed in may touch the blue toweling, and their gloved hands touch nothing outside the sterile field.

The OR is usually cold. Most of those not scrubbed—nurses, techs, residents drawn in to see this rarest of procedures—have blankets across their shoulders, draped down over their chests, giving them a rabbinical look, capped and masked, their own worlds hostile to the world telecast on the color monitors they crowd around.

"A little less talking please." Spetzler only says this when he needs maximum concentration, as now, snipping through a major membrane separating lobes of the brain along the right hemisphere, where the incision has been made. Most of the time Spetzler's OR is a chatty place; he likes it that way.

"You cannot expect 100 percent concentration and performance from everyone at all times, no matter how much you might like it," he had said. "I prefer to let people relax as much as possible, when possible, so that when the time comes that you must have 100 percent, you can demand and receive it."

Back in present tense, Spetzler's calm baritone concludes: "There should be no talking now except by those who really need to talk."

This is a critical juncture; the conversations die. South of the blue sheet, cardiac surgeon Camilla Anne Mican with her team of nurses also has been operating, inserting into the femoral artery and vein in the patient's thigh the large tubes from the giant heart-bypass pump. Possibly the highest-technology piece of equipment in the room, the pump has chrome-headed blood chambers that give it the look of a hot dragster engine; in these chambers the blood will be reoxygenated and pumped back into the patient. Developed for heart surgery in the sixties, the pump made open-heart surgery reality, then commonplace.

So far today, the heart team has been unbusy, waiting for the moment when the critical motions and decisions would be theirs. The standstill of this surgery will fall to Mican.

When hypothermic arrest was introduced for neurosurgery in the late sixties, the results were so disastrous that attempts were separated by years and involved only cases so near death that the slims odds of survival beat out the flat-zero odds of not using it.

So it had gone until a few years ago, when a handful of neurosurgeons and neuroanesthesiologists derived ever-more precise balances of barbiturates and anesthesia gases. Then they adjusted the timing of both cooling and, even more important, warming, to minimize damage to the irreplaceable brain tissue. But no surgery teams have amassed a string of successes to compare with Barrow's, today closing in on a dozen in four years. Spetzler credits the teamwork. To bring this off successfully, he says, neurosurgeons, cardiac surgeons, anesthesiologists and all manner of technicians must work in perfect concert.

But at the head of it all must be a surgeon with the skills to make use of what the technology will enable; and there are few in the country who can match Spetzler's virtuosity. The whole purpose of this massive enterprise is to provide the brain surgeon with a clear, bloodless field on which to work, for even at the high magnification of the intraoperative microscope, the tendrils of nerve and artery that might be cut while hidden in a film of blood are vital to brain function. Equally important, while the aneurysm is puffed like a balloon with blood, lifting it from its cradling brain tissue could make it rupture, and in a brain making even anesthetized demands for oxygen, that could be fatal in seconds. Now, should the aneurysm rupture, it will be in a brain with near-zero oxygen demand, and that means the rupture might be repaired before proving fatal.

In no other surgery is anesthesia so critical and thus so precisely controlled as in this. But ironically, none of it is for the purpose we most often associate with anesthesia—elimination of pain. Brain tissue feels no pain. This seat of all pleasure and pain has no sensory-nerve endings. As Spetzler works his way down, layer by layer, through neural tissue, neuroanesthesiologist Steve Shedd administers drugs that work layer by layer on consciousness. Brain activity must ultimately be damped here. Sensation of head pain can only come from the scalp, skull, cranial nerves or blood vessels, and providing analgesia, relief from pain, is the easy part of this procedure.

The cameraman from KCRA-TV, Sacramento, is perched above, on the patient's left side behind yet another curtain where neuroanesthesiologist Lisa Wilkinson watches the panels and instruments. She is assisting Shedd, who specializes in the anesthesia of hypothermic arrest and its barbiturate coma. The steady pulse-beep of the heart monitor has been so steady you don't hear it anymore, but the march of brain waves across the EEG has lessened. The EEG looks like a tide of ocean breakers that has died to a slow murmur, an outgoing tide, as the barbiturates damp all the neurons.

"We have good burst-suppression," Wilkinson says; the amplitude of the brainwaves is down low. "We have good control. Are we go?"

"Wait. We'll know in just a minute." Spetzler is adjusting the dentist's chair, forward slightly, up a notch. Everything in neurosurgery, from the chair to the microscope, must work by footpedals or mouth lever. The hands have other work. His elbows resting, Spetzler looks down through the yawning chasm he has parted, down through the Sylvian sulcus—the Valley of Sylvius—that plunges to separate the temporal lobe below from the above-aft parietal and the above-fore frontal lobes.

Fred Williams, the chief resident who had carried out earlier parts of the procedure, now stands at his left, watching through the binoculars of the second intraoperative microscope, his hands tucked under his armpits, as most of those scrubbed in do, not against the constant chill of the room, but to keep them from unsterile fields. Neurosurgeon Joseph Zabramski, assisting Spetzler, is at his right. They are frozen in tableau, these three bent over the planet. Behind them, in umpires' stance peering over shoulders, are Bruce Cherny and Paul Francis, first-year residents, and Frank Cullicchia, a fellow, his residency already completed, here for the final polish on technique, and to help teach residents. Cullicchia talks through the long afternoon with Francis and Cherny, questioning, deliberating, then falling into silence, as now, when Spetzler says, "No talking, please."

After watching the flat, two-dimensional surface glide into view and freeze on the color monitor, when you look through the intraoperative microscope the addition of depth takes your breath away. All the way down you look, through a rift a mile wide and miles deep; there is the third nerve now, a veritable rope of neuronal cables invisibly pulsing in response to the click-click-click of the audio plug in Schulte's ear. You can't see the third nerve pulse from here, but you can see it on the monitor.

And there, looming behind the third nerve, with the luster and color of pearl against the bloody field, the tip of the basilar artery balloons out with a spheroid aneurysm.

"Okay, there it is," Spetzler says. "We can't get any closer like this. Let's go."

And suddenly, the "southern" team is in motion and conversation. Spetzler pushes back, his role interrupted. He will leave surgeries in progress for periods as long as half an hour, returning to check on progress. Now everyone on the cardiac team is at something. Mican and her assistant hunch over the femoral artery in the patient's leg; the heart-pump technician spins dials and switches. Soon bright blood courses through the clear plastic hose, fills the machine's shiny-topped cannisters, and courses back out again. This is all that appears to be happening, but what a sea change goes on inside the man.

The bypass machine is refrigerating the blood, little by little, before sending it homeward. And periodically over the next hour, one voice or another will read the brain temperature monitor: "33 degrees" centigrade, meaning 91.4 Fahrenheit, seven degrees below normal. Then "31," and "29," all the way down to 23 degrees, or 73.4 degrees Fahrenheit.

And then a jolt of potassium chloride to the heart stops it from beating.

Beeeee! The final beep of the heart monitor draws out endlessly, in alarm. Mican is now in complete control of Schulte's circulation, through the heart pump; in the deepening chill, some blood is still being pumped to his ever-quieting brain. "19 degrees," Wilkinson reports, 66.2 Fahrenheit, well below even this room's temperature. The brain normally could not stand this cold; its neurons would die. But the bypass pumps and chills onward.

Spetzler, at the illuminated wall, talks with Williams and Zabramski. "Z" had been a resident of Spetzler's at Case Western Reserve, Spetzler's last post. He had come here with the Boss, becoming chief resident two years earlier, then got that highest accolade the director could give: He was hired. Zabramski was the ninth and newest member of the neurosurgical team at Barrow, making it one of the larger such neuro staffs in the country.

They wait for Jack Schulte's temperature to drop, but the wait is not a quiet one. Every few minutes, it seems, either Tom Grahm or another resident comes through the door, clutching x-rays, CTs, MRI scans, which they splay against the lighted wall, crack, crack, crack. There is a lot of hurried pointing, questioning from Spetzler, and out they go again.

What's up?

"Something about a kid hit by a car. In real bad shape. They thought at first he was neurologically intact, but now he's going down."

By 4 p.m., seven hours after opening, Schulte's brain was damping down to the limit it could be taken. It was time. The blood still pumps through the patient, then through the refrigerator-pump, and back again. Body temperature 16.1 centigrade—just under 61 degrees Fahrenheit. Brain 17 degrees, just under 63 Fahrenheit. The brain always lags behind, because its own tissue warms the blood in all those thousands of roothair branch points.

Zabramski explains that many failures with hypothermic arrest in the past occurred because brain and body temperature were assumed the same, so blood-pumping was being stopped at too warm a temperature for the brain, a temperature at which it was still carrying out vital functions, requiring oxygen.

At this point, with brain temperature just below 63 degrees, Spetzler says quietly, "Stop altogether."

"Doing it."

The pump technician says: "Pumps off at ten after the hour" of 4 p.m.

"I would like only those people to talk who really need to talk," Spetzler says quietly. "Are we counting down?"

"All drained," Mican says.

And there you have it. A brain as cold and quiet as the grave.

What does that mean, inside? Imagine cranking up the intraoperative microscope from its maximum 35 times, to 1,000 power, so a field of neurons would occupy the stage, and we could watch them live, metabolizing, signalling, taking in oxygen, giving off carbon dioxide.

The neuron is *the* brain cell, and must be the focus again and again in trying to understand how the "machinery" of the conscious self works. All the other cells of the brain serve to support neurons in one way or another.

Animal cells have more in common than not, as though one prototype cell were modified so that parts could be bent or extended or shrunk to fit particular jobs. And since we all begin as single fertilized eggs, in many ways that's exactly what cell differentiation is all about.

One of the major qualities that differentiates animal cell types is how long they live. Skin cells live only about ninety days, red blood cells about the same, though some of the marrow cells that produce blood are replaced every few hours. They are constantly replenished throughout life. By contrast, the neurons of the brain grow with unbelievable rapidity during fetal development.

In just under nine months, the first neuron precursor cells become 100 billion. And then right around birth they come to an absolute stop, a suddenness unmatched in the formation of other organs. Unless something goes awry, in an especially rare form of brain cancer, these brain cells never grow again. A newborn baby has all the neurons it ever will.

Luckily, only a tiny percentage of these cells is ever needed, and in some circumstances throughout life dead neurons are replaced by standbys. How that is possible is mysterious now—as it becomes better known, better recovery from stroke and traumatic cell death may be achieved. But if all the brain is present at birth, what's missing? A newborn baby plainly is not "neurologically intact;" in fact, many of its reflex motions, such as flexing and extending limbs and sucking are the mark of severe coma in adults.

Connections are missing. And more connections. And connections among the already-connected. MIT's Walle Nauta, one of the world's leading neuro-anatomists, pointed out that some single motor cells, which send their signaling "wires" to muscle fibers, have as many as 10,000 receptors getting inputs from other neurons. And how many receptors might there be to each of those 10,000? Even if you imagine that each of those signalling cells was getting input from only 1,000 others, the number of "inputs" just at that second level would be 10 million, without going to the number of inputs *those* cells had. But for what we're after all these are meaningless numbers, because many of the signaling cells we're talking about are communicating with *one another,* forming loops that both inhibit and enhance the firing off of new signals.

As if this exponential growth in connection were not complexity enough, Nauta noted, recent investigations indicate that neuroanatomists may have miscounted the sheer numbers of neurons by two orders of magnitude. He believes there actually may be 10 trillion, not 100 billion. As some indication of the scope of such an increase—using 100 billion as the number of neurons—biologists estimate adults to average 10 trillion *total* cells. For the sake of consistency with other writings, let's consider 100 billion the average human's neuronal complement, especially because the true measure of brain power appears to be not mass, but connections.

This virtually endless interconnectivity proves only that you cannot under-stand how the brain works by following the cell to cell wiring, just as you could not understand America by calculating with which and with how many individuals each individual communicates. Some communications are more frequent or intense, some less, some merely potential. But in both cases, we can see that communication and relationship is what the higher level of meaning is all about. *Connections* among the brain cells grow explosively as babies develop into children, adolescents into adults, and adults' brain-cell connections modify continually, if less explosively, for as long as they live.

How do neurons communicate? Electrically, and in a way that is schematically easy to understand. A typical neuron is large—so large that a single one of the largest variety would be about the size of a dust mote—visible to the naked eye, if you knew what you were looking at. The cell body has a tangle of incoming roots, called dendrites, and a single long outgoing projection, called an axon. Electric signals from other neurons come in through the dendrites and add up arithmetically as they roll toward the axon "gateway." If the charge adds enough to open the gate, then an electric burst is sent outward on the axon. That pulse thrums at a constant voltage along the entire length of this axonal wire, to as many branch spots as the cell communicates with. The pulse of one single neuron is relatively powerful—sometimes as high as half a volt. And the thrumming of billions of neurons in synchrony, like the roar of ocean waves or—a better analogy—the mixed pitches and frequencies of waves in the air that define the playing of music, add up to our brain waves. Specific sets of these are monitored on an electroencephalogram, or EEG, just as the percussion section of an orchestra could be picked out of a symphony.

So what is brain death? Not the death of all neurons, but the end of their communication. The end of the empire of the mind comes long before most of its citizens have died. It may take days for the last neuron in a dead person's brain to die, just as it takes days before the last cells of the rest of the body die, and potentially years before they all decompose. But at some early point, communication ends and death is irreversible.

That is why this standstill occupies such a mysterious territory. The chilled neurons are receiving no oxygen and no nutrients; there is no blood to deliver them; the only new oxygen coming in is from residual blood left behind in tissues. What the lowered temperature means when translated into cellular metabolism is that there is radically less metabolism going on. Temperature to a scientist is a measure of energy in a system, and this system normally operates only at an energy-level corresponding to 98.6 degrees Fahrenheit, give or take a couple of degrees of fever.

Look at one brain cell. At 63 degrees Fahrenheit, and further dampened by barbiturates and the stillness of anesthesia, it is using less than half the energy it did when Schulte was awake and thinking. Further, the neuron uses by far most of its energy to send out that powerful electrical pulse, the requirement of consciousness and the constant activity that *is* "brain life." This neuron is not pulsing. Therefore it can use the energy stored within to maintain itself. But not for long. Not so far, in neurosurgery. Within an hour, pulse or no pulse, the cell will begin to suffocate without new oxygen, which it needs even more than nutrients. And once a cell truly begins to die, it dies fast.

Still, there is no communication going on among these brain cells. So the standstill brings a hope that seems as easy to fulfill as the alchemist's wish to transmute lead into gold, that physicians could "suspend animation" indefinitely. The brain waves that are the mark of brain life have been suspended, just as in death.

But suspended animation may prove even more elusive than the creation of gold, because this picture of the quiet cell lacks resolution. Despite appearances now, within each of Jack Schulte's brain cells the fire of metabolism, though banked, burns on. To literally suspend animation would require that, for an indefinite period, you could freeze every brain cell down to the molecular level, to prevent the breakdown of molecules, to prevent the formation of new ones needing much lower energy levels to maintain them. Freezing molecules is not just one analogous step down from freezing meat, because to a scientist freezing at that level means lowering energy and implies a breakdown of high-energy molecules into low-energy ones. A tough mountain to get over to get to that alluring *what if.* But tantalizingly thinkable, especially looking at these monitors here in OR 1. Quiet as death.

Back Spetzler plunges, braced against the binoculars of the microscope as the monitor shows us the canyon down through the Sylvian valley, past the third nerve. But there is a world of difference now. We are looking at a white moonscape, a clear bloodless field where the giant aneurysm stands out pearl against alabaster, and tiny perforator arteries can be seen against the basilar artery as Spetzler follows it, lifeline, to the swelling.

He tugs, pries, gently with the two critical instruments of neurosurgery, the scalpel and the Malis bipolar cautery. The cautery resembles a giant pair of electrified tweezers. When its twin prongs close down on conductive brain tissue, a micro current flows between the prongs, searing the tissue to prevent bleeding from the many tiny but vital blood vessels in any portion of brain tissue.

As Spetzler asks for adjustment of the electric current upward and downward, a computerized voice with a curiously New York accent replies, "Twenty-five, twenty-five, twenty-five," or "Thirty, thirty, thirty." Curious, perhaps, but not accidental. It is the voice of Leonard Malis, pioneer in microneurosurgery and inventor of the cautery, frozen on a computer chip.

Cautery and knife move slowly even at this magnification. And then Spetzler is there; his dissector blade is right at the aneurysm.

"How many minutes?"

"Three."

Pam Smith, the audiovisual technician who videotapes and photographs key procedures for presentations, publications, grand rounds for hospital personnel, has from time to time climbed her rolling stepladder to shoot from above. Now Spetzler wants some still photos through the intraoperative microscope, tells her so even as he works downward, his voice disembodied. In fact the voice's rhythm is so different from the hands' that they seem to belong to two different people, with two different sets of concerns on the mission.

"Shoot!" He orders, and Smith replies, "No moving." For perhaps two seconds the moonscape vanishes from the monitor as the still camera rotates into position, under her guidance through foot pedals, then rotates back again, the moonscape returning.

Spetzler loads a clip into the applicator pliers that hold it apart. Virtually every object of use in the operating room, no matter how homely in appearance, is the product of intensive, purposeful development, and the clip-applicator is no exception. The Yasargil 9-mm clip Spetzler will use to tie off the aneurysm is a "V" of steel with a spring neck at the base. It is held open by special pliers with long, slender handles, rotated into position and precisely released to place the clip. Likewise, the working of virtually every piece of high-technology equipment in here requires intensive training and exceptional manual dexterity.

Spetzler now attempts to set the clip's jaws around the bulb of the aneurysm. "Shoot."

"No moving."

Vanish, return; vanish, return. The clip still is not set; he has gotten it around the neck of the aneurysm, but each time he lets the jaws close down, some of the aneurysm slips free. Finally, he sets the clip. It is four-fifteen, five minutes into arrest, but seems much longer. But Spetzler does not like the clip's position, withdraws it and tries again.

"How many minutes?"

"Eleven."

He retracts, suctions, tugs away perforators, tiny even under the microscope, from where they adhere to the side of the huge artery, and resumes trying to reseat the clip. As often as he succeeds he removes it. He says, "Ah, look now, almost perfect."

One of his scrub nurses remarks, "You can always tell when he says 'almost perfect' that he's going to try again."

Now the clip is seated again. Spetzler is finally satisfied with its placement; but there is no tone of triumph, no mark that this is the climactic moment, for all he says is, "How long, please?"

"18 minutes."

"Start the pump please."

"We're back on bypass."

And that is the moment. Jack Schulte's little death ends at four twenty-eight. Hopefully. Blood wells up through the surgical incision, but no cause for alarm. Resident Paul Francis says, "It's diffuse, coming from everywhere. It'll drain." Schulte's blood has been treated with the drug heparin, so that whatever remained after the draining would not clot, and so it will tend to squeeze out of even the tiniest blood vessels.

Suddenly, the signal returns to the EEG monitor. The dance of the neurons resumes.

"Would you send word to the family that all is going satisfactorily," Spetzler says. A nurse takes the phone, steps outside the operating room door.

Schulte is still on bypass. His heart has not yet started, though with the resumption of blood flow through the heart, body and brain, Mican now detects some fibrillation of the heart muscle. Though regulated by the brain, the heart will beat on its own, its nerves sending direct signals to the smooth-muscle cells to contract.

It is four forty-five now and body temperature is high enough that the heart can be restarted. Mican's nurse holds two electric shock pads over Schulte's chest.

"All clear?"

All monitors now must be disconnected or be fried as the electricity hits the heart.

"Clear."

A jolt; the drapery leaps as the chest heaves under the shock. Then nothing.

"Clear!"

Jolt. The drapery leaps again.

"*Nada,*" someone says.

What will happen if the heart does not start? Mican will open Schulte's chest, just as fast as she can, and attempt to restart it by massage.

"Clear!"

Jolt.

"All right!" The voice is from anesthesia, where Wilkinson's expert ear has picked up a most-welcome sound: the steady click, click, click of a heart monitor.

Plunged deep in a coma where he is expected, at best, to remain for days, Jack Schulte is, in every sense of the word, alive again.

The heart pump will remain connected for another half hour as blood pressure rebuilds, and Fred Williams will not begin the slow, tedious process of closing until blood pressure is restored and normal clotting can be achieved. They must know before closing that no new hemorrhage is breaking out. But at five-thiry, they are near the end of a road that had begun before ten.

Once the closing is begun and Schulte is out of immediate danger, Spetzler peels off his gloves, "scrubbing out," and as always says to the crew, "Thank you very much, everyone."

Spetzler's Luck

SPETZLER QUICKLY UNWRAPS his surgeon's gown, leaving him in the standard hospital uniform of blue-linen scrubs—short-sleeved pullover blouse and string-tied trousers. Like most of his peers, he leads an intensely-athletic "leisure" life, his arms still tanned from a week's snorkeling trip to the Caribbean two months ago, to which he had jetted from a neurosurgery ski meeting in Colorado. He pulls the blue-paper cap back from a thick shock of brown hair as he exits the OR and snaps off his mask, revealing a clipped mustache that tends to jut slightly above his full mouth.

Leaning against the wall in the hallway, he says, "I feel it went very well." There is a touch of exhilaration in his voice, but, characteristically, little inflection. "And it was a case that would have had a devastating outcome without hypothermic arrest. You saw me pulling tiny blood vessels away from the dome of the aneurysm. That would not have been possible unless the dome was collapsed" by the draining of its blood supply. "If I'd included those perforators in the clip, they would have certainly led to stroke in the brain-stem area."

He speaks slowly and thoughtfully, weighing his words when he is most caught up in the importance of a subject, his voice deep but usually without animation. And that carries over to his facial expressions. He is a man of few mannerisms of any sort and when he is most intent, as now in mid-conversation, he tends to stare fixedly into middle distance. The closest to absentmindedness or carelessness of movement you will find is his occasionally twisting his mustache as he talks or thinks.

He wastes no motion. Nearly all the OR personnel tie their face masks in quick bows. Spetzler knots his, half-a-beat quicker, then breaks the tie with a quick snap when he's done. Everyone else wears paper booties over their shoes, more to protect the shoes from blood than the floor from shoes. The Boss wears one of three identical pairs of ivory-colored leather loafers, silicone-treated and thus washable. No booties. Trifling, but an unnecessary spending of time.

All these characteristics are subtle, the sort of things you notice only after you know who he is. But here in the hospital, walking alone, among nurses in the OR, among his residents during his daily rounds, even among colleagues here or in informal settings, there is nothing about his manner that would lead you to suspect that he is among the very best in the world at what he does. Nor is there anything that marks him as arrogant. He is unfailingly polite and never condescending or brittle. He has a quick wit and a ready smile, although among his crew the wit shows in affection rather than broader humor.

Peers determine one's ranking in stature and arrogance, and Spetzler gets ranked near the top in both by them, but it is important to consider who they are. Brain surgeons are the elite of the medical world in the popular imagination, so much so that it's hardly surprising that they see themselves that way. After all, they saw through that popular lens when they dreamed youthful dreams of what they would be. One way or another their personalities show the depth of that belief. Every competition is pursued with an air of camaraderie that belies a deadly earnestness. Every instrument is mastered; there are no toys, only tools. Every endeavor is pursued with complete intensity.

Bennett Stein, chair at Columbia and Spetzler's longtime friend, says, "We're all a bunch of wild men and egomaniacs."

And vascular neurosurgeons see themselves as the elite of that breed, practitioners of the hardest art in the hardest place to practice on the hardest structures to resolve found on earth. Into that company, Spetzler thrust himself.

In high school he knew he would be a neurosurgeon. By the time he was in medical school he knew he would be a vascular neurosurgeon. It was the difficulty that drew him. The precision and intensity. "The brain, after all, is the ultimate organ. And the vascular system the most challenging, the most unforgiving of error. When I was in residency, if you could do vascular neurosurgery, then that's what you did."

In his mid-forties on this April day, he was already very near the pinnacle of world neurosurgery. The standstills were not the only reason, or even the major reason. They were the high-tech, brilliant "miracle surgeries" that drew attention to him and showcased his talent. They were not a legacy, and if you were at the top, there was one thing beyond your standing to become obsessed with, the final peak: a legacy. What mark would you leave on world neurosurgery in a career, as he was fond of saying, that is half a career. If you were very good and very lucky, as Spetzler was, you became a chairman young, in your early forties, a time when professional athletes were retired and people in most other physically-demanding professions were at or past the pinnacle of their careers.

By the time you became a chairman of a major neurological institute, you couldn't help but already be thinking of what your career might ultimately mean. "Ultimate" in medicine is easy to state as a generalization: You trained the next generation of top specialists in your field. What that might mean in particular was harder to state, but you could glean it over time, in complex and subtle ways. Spetzler was complex and subtle. His residents and fellows saw it, dimly at first; they all began, right in the initial interview process, in awe of his beguiling and friendly manner, as though he were laying a trap. He was not; he is not an easy man to know, but he lets himself be known.

One of his residents tellingly observed, "He's very friendly and approachable, but sometimes he seems aloof, in another world. I think he is in another world, but he wants you to see it, too."

Spetzler's raw talents are as easy to portray as any super-athlete's. They showed plainly in the Schulte surgery; they would be showcased over the next three days as never before or for some years after. He can reach into areas of the brain where only a few others can reach without damage, because his physical coordination is superb.

Setting a Yasargil aneurysm clip, for example, requires the surgeon to hold a pair of long-handled pliers in one hand, six inches or more above the small aneurysm deep within the cavity he has created, and to be steady enough to keep the far end of this wand, which holds the clip open, from wavering. Then, from this height, he must rotate the wrist clockwise or counterclockwise until the clip aligns with the longitude of the bulbed-out artery or vein. When alignment is just so, gently release and the clip closes down, sealing the balloon off from the still-firm vascular tubing. And if that position is not "just so," then the clip must be reseated in the pliers' nose, opened wide, tried again.

Someone with such skills, as he says, can attempt surgeries that others cannot. But he has a far deeper and more complex brain-skill than good hand-eye coordination. He has an ability to project in three dimensions so acute that going from MRI and CT scans and angiograms to the table, he always knows precisely where he is. He sees what is beyond the layer of tissue facing him.

A resident says, "A lot of really great neurosurgeons always operate from a particular side, like the left, or even from one specific position on the left, because that's where they see things best, that's their point of reference. But Spetzler stands everywhere and anywhere; it doesn't matter. He sees just as well from any angle."

The skill he works hardest to teach his residents during their daily "Spetzler rounds" is to see real structures where only flat scans appear. Not just to imagine or think about a structure but see precisely where it lies in relation to the structure you now are parting with blade, scissors, or electric cautery. The structure might be a tiny bundle of nerves meaning vision, hearing, motion; it might be a tiny artery all but invisible in a film of blood, feeding a small cluster of cells virtually indistinguishable from others but controlling the ability to speak language rather than make vocal noises, to understand verbs, to recognize faces as more than shapes, to lay down new memories of any kind.

And for each structure, there is a distinctive web of blood vessels. Here is the vascular neurosurgeon's territory.

The brain's arteries, looking like skeletons of tumbleweed or any other fan-shaped bush stripped by winter, rise from a few sturdy stalks, rapidly branching and ending in wisps. The scans show them in two-dimensional projections; therefore a slight brightening of artery or vein usually means it has changed direction from the flat plane and is now headed out of the scan toward you or down and away from you, so you are looking end-on at a cylinder. Sometimes so slight a brightening means the balloon of an aneurysm whose rupture would mean stroke.

How do you come to an understanding of that complex of webbing? Learning so that as you work down through brain tissue and see a tiny purple tube, you know if it's an artery or part of that mirror network, the veinous drainage, and if it's an artery, to what vital brain area it is delivering blood—all brain areas are vital, but some are more so.

In the strictest sense of vital, essential to life, no blood supply is more important than that supplying the brain stem, in whose three major divisions the controls of life are seated, and it is along the brain stem that the major feeders of the brain's blood supply arise. Like finding your way around a city by studying the major freeways on a map and noting where they branch, starting at the great arteries at the base of the brain is the easiest way to get into this six-inch hemispheroid planet, flattened fore where it rests on the skull shelf just above the eyes.

The left and right vertebral arteries climb the front of the lowest segment of brain stem, the medulla oblongata. At the top of the medulla, the vertebrals join to form the basilar artery just as the medulla swells into the much larger middle segment, the pons, or bridge. The major hemispheres of the brain—what we think of when we picture a brain—are pushed down like a mushroom cap over the third and uppermost section of brain stem, the diencephalon, the highest level of "generically-animal" brain.

The basilar artery runs along the front of the pons. From it branch left and right versions of four separate arteries supplying the cerebellum, two at the lower end of the basilar, two at the top; and between those sets of cerebellar arteries are three arteries suppling the pons itself. The basilar artery is also as remote from the surface as any part of the brain, running its course near the center of this Earth. A vital structure in the center of the brain: That offers some idea why damage to the basilar artery is usually swiftly fatal, and why aneurysms there are among the most difficult for the neurosurgeon to reach and to treat.

Just as the basilar artery reaches the underside of the mushroom cap hemispheres, it enters a blood-routing network to rival any urban traffic circle, and it looks like one. It is the major vascular complex of the skull base.

To get a rough idea how the complex of the upper brain is supplied, put your wrists together, cupping your hands upwards, fingers splayed, as a child does when learning to catch a ball. Now the fingers rise like arteries, the heels of your hands forming a rough circle. That is the circle of Willis. From the circle of Willis most of the major cerebral thoroughfares take off. The basilar artery enters the circle of Willis from below, at the rear. Just over halfway around, on the left and right, the internal carotid arteries enter from below. These three are the major suppliers of blood through the circle.

This is one of the few places in the body where blood travels in a circle, and that is one of the brain's major safety mechanisms. If the supply from either side is interrupted, blood from the other side, called collateral blood flow, can help make up the loss. One person's ability to survive loss of a brain blood vessel without permanent damage while another is crippled or killed is often the difference between the strength of their collateral blood flow, but it is a difference virtually impossible to estimate.

From the circle of Willis, at the point nearest the basilar artery, the posterior cerebral arteries arise to branch throughout the huge upper cerebrum. At the frontal side the anterior cerebral arteries arise out of the middle cerebral arteries. Between the two anterior cerebral arteries runs the anterior communicating artery, "A-Com," in neurosurgeon's parlance. The circle is completed at the rear, just after the basilar artery splits into the posterior cerebral arteries, by the posterior communicating artery, "P-Com," which links posterior cerebral with middle cerebral arteries.

But that offers only a hint of the generic complexity of the neurovascular system. There is a whole new level of complexity, very easy to summarize for those who do not need to understand it in enough detail to deal with it. Human arteries and veins also grow and develop with a remarkable *individual* variation. Not only the smaller branches but even the major feeders show surprising variations in position and branch-point within the normal range, everywhere in the body. For example, although we think of the body as a left-right mirror image, the left and right common-carotid arteries can come off the heart and branch in several entirely different ways, and they can even arise from different trunk lines. Which pattern your common carotids follow depends on family inheritance, but all the variations function perfectly normally.

Vascularization of the brain in the embryo is much the same. Arteries are sent invading tissue in lock-step with the tissues' growing demand for blood, and as long as enough blood gets where it is needed and can meet fluctuating demands, many variations work. This is an important fact about vascularization. In embryonic development, growth of blood vessels is only partly a response to genetic instructions. It is also a response to demand.

So once vascular neurosurgeons have memorized all the names and branch points of the arteries and veins, and seen just what they look like from every angle in two-dimensional projection, then on the days before this next surgery there must be the intense scrutiny, *de novo*: scans of this brain, to press into their own brains the image of where the branchings and turnings are in this brain—the one that will be under the cautery tomorrow.

These are consummate intellectual puzzles, to which neurosurgeons bring consummate hands-on solutions, but "hands-on" captures little of what drives any surgeon. Dedication and training are higher order of mental activity, like motivation. But the desire and drive that are central in all those who use "the healing blade" are basic, culminating in the visceral thrill all surgeons experience by taking procedures to the edge. The phrase "the healing blade" itself has nuances that show the surgeon becoming wedded to the craft. Overtly it is used with mock-seriousness, as in, "This looks like a case for the healing blade." But ultimately the joke becomes a mask for the passionate belief. And there is a less romantic way of looking at where this leads. The further surgeons can push the limits of the surgery, the bigger the thrill, both immediately, from the difficult physical manipulations, and long term if they outdistance their surgical rivals. Surgeons are famous among physicians for "loving to cut," and they stand out among those in the competitive medical professions for loving to lord it over their rivals.

And this unromantic side to surgeons shows powerfully in the politics of surgery. There are more good surgeons in all subspecialties than good positions. Competition is intense. Frequently promotions are based on personalities more than abilities, just as in business, politics, or other fields of endeavor.

Personal animosities can infect professional relationships and ruin careers.

Consummately skilled, consummately driven; that tells much about who neurosurgeons are as a group, but of course very little about who each man and woman is, or how this one got to where we find him on a day of remarkably early heat in a city in the Sonoran Desert.

ROBERT FRIEDERICH SPETZLER was born Nov. 13, 1944 in a small town near Würzburg, Germany, the third of six children of August and Maria Spetzler. The Spetzler family was renowned for its engineering skill, and August was prosperous enough to weather the depression and Second World War with less financial trauma than many.

But it was a dangerous time to stand out from the crowd. When the bomb-plot against Hitler surfaced, August and a cousin fell under suspicion as possible designers of the timing mechanism. August was then in combat on the Russian front. His civilian cousin was dragged from his home by the Gestapo and, in front of his wife and children, shot to death as a conspirator. Although wounded in combat, August recovered. He never spoke to his children about any of this until he reached his eightieth birthday. All that the Spetzler children knew of that period was that their father hated weapons; even after they emigrated to America, when Robert was nine, they were not allowed to play cowboys and Indians—not that six siblings lacked for other action or mischief.

But the keystone experience of Robert Spetzler's childhood had already occurred before they left Germany, at age five, a time from which he dates his entire life. He barely remembers anything before it. Ultra-vivid memories began then.

Robert cut his foot, whether on a rusty nail or rock, he can't remember. He developed tetanus, a muscular disease caused by infection of spores from the soil-dwelling *Clostridium* bacteria, which secrete neurotoxins. The toxins attack the motor nerves that directly control muscles. Tetanus refers to a muscular tensing that follows instantly on an earlier tensing, a short-circuit of stimulation. The affected muscles are in constant and uncontrollable spasm. The toxins first strike the muscles controlling the jaw, causing it to gnash and tear the tongue, then to paralyze the jaw locked. Eventually the toxins attack the nerves controlling the diaphragm until tetanus paralyzes its muscles, causing death by suffocation.

Robert was placed in a storage room, where iron lungs were kept. "They were absolutely certain I would die, and they didn't want me out with the other children," he says evenly, "where my death would upset them." He recalls his mother's face, pale and distraught, pressed against the observation glass daily.

He did not die partly because he was one of the first German tetanus victims to receive penicillin, a secret Allied drug during the war that now made its way into Germany. Penicillin kills the spores that produce the toxin, but only time can remove the toxin itself from the system. He spent a long period near death, and luck was at least partly responsible for his survival.

But it was not that experience that decided him on becoming a doctor. "No, no indeed. I remember being taken as an example of someone who had tetanus and survived, taken in front of a big auditorium where there were a lot of medical students. I was not treated with warmth at the hospital. I was just presented as an interesting case. It was a very negative experience." The broad, confident smile now, somewhat conspiratorial. It is one of the few gestures with which he gives himself away, of course deliberately: "It gave me a lot of attention, being a sibling in the middle of six children."

The family emigrated a few years later, when August lost his business after a partner fled with its assets. At nine, Robert was still young enough to lose all but the trace of an accent. Negative introduction to medicine or no, by the time he signed off on his high school yearbook in suburban Illinois, Spetzler declared that he would become a brain surgeon. He can't remember now how or when he knew.

But something happened in between, in his adolescence, that he does remember clearly, that shaped and for the first time truly focused his energies, surprising in its power, foreshadowing his adult character.

If you ask those closest to him at Barrow what Spetzler's major gifts are, after they mention the physical skills there is a pause. He is well-focused and well-organized, they say. Invariably the neurosurgeon or fellow or resident stops there, realizing this sounds inadequate. Only Peter Raudzens, the head of neuroanesthesia, plunges ahead, clear on the import of what this means. "R" is Spetzler's sidekick in tension-breaking adventures, glacier skiing in British Columbia, scuba diving in the Caribbean. "R" understands this about the Boss.

"He is not merely organized; he is so completely organized on so many levels that he appears to be doing several things at once, if you don't know him. If you know him, you know he does only one thing at a time on which his concentration, his focus, is absolute."

Total focus certainly is a magnificent gift for a neurosurgeon. But the ability to change focus abruptly, to keep many vitally important projects going at once, is a gift for the director. And there is something else, harder to put but, to Raudzens, as real: Spetzler has a reputation for being lucky, and just when you think that luck isn't part of the formula in neurosurgery, something happens to make you wonder if serendipity does not play some role here. When the odds are even, things tend to fall Spetzler's way; Raudzens lays that off to focus, to results of it that cannot be clearly seen, such as to preparations more exhaustive than they appear.

Regardless of its value, Spetzler says that focus was not innate but a quality he developed fairly late. "I was fairly unfocused in grade school and high school, except for projects which interested me. And if something interested me, then I threw my entire energy into it."

By the time Spetzler was in high school, he had been studying piano for half a dozen years, but was not particularly devoted to it. Then midway through high school he wanted something, so passionately that he *had* to have it, and that helped make him the excellent musician he is.

He wanted a horse.

August Spetzler was far from wealthy, and in any event did not believe in supporting his children beyond the necessities; family income certainly would not provide for anything as outlandish as a horse.

Within weeks of knowing he had to have a horse, Robert was working three jobs while going to high school. He gave piano lessons and tuned pianos, jobs that would have been otherwise boring but which paid far better wages than a teenager could earn any other way. At night he worked as a hospital orderly, but not because he had any interest in medicine.

He wanted not just a horse but an unbroken horse. That's what he bought, a horse no one had been able to ride. Bought it, climbed on top, got thrown off. Got thrown off more times than he could count; finally mastered it. Far from disapproving of his son's wild notion, August enthusiastically followed, as did several of the others. Soon the Spetzlers had rented land from a farmer on which they built their own horse barn; soon each owned an unbroken horse, and that became the family's sport, training unbroken horses. Not for show or for breeding—although Robert did breed Lady and raised her foal. Just for the pleasure of Western-saddle riding on horses they had broken and trained themselves.

He studied biology at Knox College, where he lettered in swimming and graduated *cum laude* with honors in biology. And the good fortune of knowing he wanted to be a neurosurgeon gave him a competitive edge over his classmates. "When I did an honors biology project, it was on circulation in the brain. In medical school, I don't think I was better than many others, but I never missed a neurosurgery or neurology conference."

He chose Northwestern for his medical training, because neurosurgery was headed by Paul Bucy, who had trained with the great Harvey Cushing and gone on to become one of America's great teachers himself, to Spetzler the greatest.

So confident was Bucy in the future of his protégé that he sent Spetzler as a medical student to Zurich, to study under another of the great names in world neurosurgery, Gazi Yasargil, inventor of the clip Spetzler had just placed on Schulte and which, its size and simplicity notwithstanding, had saved hundreds of lives from death by stroke in the rupture of aneurysms.

Spetzler returned from Europe to find Northwestern in turmoil, because Bucy was planning retirement. But this first mentor presented him a list of the top residency programs in the country with a promise to help him get where he wanted. At the top of Bucy's list was the University of California at San Francisco, where young Charles Wilson was building what was being called the nation's top neurosurgical training program. Spetzler picked it without hesitation.

And Robert became Charlie's star. Not just then, but for years after. Other Wilson graduates had to listen—perhaps too frequently—to lines that went, "That's not the way Robert would do it." Or, "Robert could already do this by the end of his second year."

It was wild horses all over again. Not right away, even under the legendarily-demanding Wilson, not until near the end of his residency, he says. But finally, he knew. "It became obvious I was fortunate to have chanced upon my profession and my passion in the same place, in surgery, in the brain. I always knew I wanted neurosurgery, but I did not know I had the focus to spend all my free time and energy on this."

So dryly put it might have been a conclusion drawn in the middle of a committee meeting, the kind Spetzler hates, involving pallid issues like the politics of neurosurgery. But once, earlier, when he was asked if there was any single moment in his training that defined him, Spetzler replied without hesitation:

"I was chief resident at the VA Hospital in San Francisco, a chief residency you get before your final year of training. I was opening a closed skull fracture in which all the indications were that no bleeding had occurred. Charlie Wilson was at my side but he was not scrubbed in." A pause while you absorb that. Wilson could not take over for him.

Suddenly blood came pouring out, from everywhere at once it seemed. "I was in trouble. But Charlie had confidence in me, that I could get out of trouble. And I got myself out of trouble." Surprise, the deepest dread in this most-carefully rehearsed and choreographed of medical specialties, had come at him from everywhere, and he had met and bested it.

That night, he dreamed. He was studying the scans again and saw no indication of bleeding, nor did Wilson. Now he opened and blood came rushing at him, and he woke. He lay awake thinking about what he might have done differently. But no, all the indications were that no brain bleeding had occurred. He had done right and could sleep now, and so he drifted down until he was there again and suddenly ....That was the first time Spetzler remembers the big nightmare. But then when he finally woke up, he knew. *Charlie had confidence in me ... and I got myself out of trouble.*

Suddenly the diverse world snaps into singularity, not because it is one-dimensional but just the opposite, because it can be seen as one from any angle. Everything is connected. It is now possible to waste no motion. It is now possible to waste no time.

Spetzler is near the pinnacle, but that is not enough. Barrow is not yet near the pinnacle. The legacy is not just in performing the impossible neurosurgery for the first time, where no one has the skill or the confidence to go. He had to be chairman of the best neurological institute in America. That did not mean it would not have peers, but that no place would be ahead of its few peers. Barrow was not there, not this April, and so he was not there.

What does it take for an institution to be at the top? The judgment of the director's peers, for one, and they have to be the directors of peer institutions, passing a judgment based on factors as complex as those going into understanding and evaluating an individual.

For the institute, too, there must be a focus. This is a neurological institute, where the neuro arts must not be second-string appendages of other branches of medicine. But just as with an individual, the singular focus must not be a mark of one-dimensionality, and that was Barrow's flaw now. As a neurosurgical institute—Spetzler believed—it had few peers and no betters. But as a research institution, it had one glaring weakness, and that was in neurology. Neurology was not nationally competitive.

Charlie Wilson had warned him he would come to this place in his life. Brilliant and charismatic, Robert was also notorious for popping off, at conferences and elsewhere, about ways his predecessors did things that could use improvement—predecessors who were alive, well, practicing, and sitting in the room as he spoke.

Classic case in point, and not a single occurrence but a series of events with a much wider and more august audience than even a major conference would provide. Spetzler was just six years out of residency, 39 years old and an assistant professor at Case Western Reserve, when its director, Frank Nelson, retired. Spetzler thought he was the logical choice to succeed him as director of this top neurosurgery program. Robert Ratcheson, Spetzler's senior, was the choice. Spetzler did not take it well.

Bad blood is said to remain between Ratcheson and Spetzler, although Spetzler insists, "At no time was I impolite or rude. That just is not my style." But Wilson, who thinks Spetzler is "absolutely first rate, a crackerjack, one of the best in the world," says, "Robert was not a good sport about that, no question about it."

Reminded of that, Spetzler breaks into an eager, wiseguy grin. "Let's put it this way. I was way too young to think of myself so seriously for that job. And not having gotten it, I definitely should have kept my mouth shut. I definitely should not have written a letter to the search committee."

Spetzler told the search committee—like all such committees culled from among the top neurosurgeons in the country—that he had wanted to make Case the best institution in the country by giving it the best neurosurgery training program. Too bad. "Now I'll have to create the best training program somewhere else," he said.

John Green had come calling, looking for an heir to head Barrow Neurological Institute in Phoenix. So be it.

Wilson's advice was unequivocal as ever. "I said, 'Robert, for God's sake, the place is a wasteland! You'll die out there. Bide your time and wait for the chairmanship of a top institute to come your way.' But Robert was on the rebound and he was going to show them all."

And would still pop off while doing it. Here was a rising star of the new generation of neurosurgeons, heading an institute shouldering to the front in terms of the number of neurosurgical procedures and its outpouring of publications, but he lacked what many felt was sufficient respect for those of arguably greater eminence—or, inarguably, of longer-standing eminence.

These are the kinds of failings that have little effect on the surgical achievements of one with Spetzler's skills. But in the wider world outside the operating room, they can have telling effects on one's advancement up the ever-narrowing pyramid of chairmanships at ever-more elite neurosurgical institutes, or of presidencies of the most important neurosurgical groups, and virtually all of those who have reached Spetzler's level have their eyes on their final place in the firmament. He does.

Spetzler makes no bones about his outspokenness. "I have never held my tongue when I felt someone's presentation was not what it should have been just because of the presenter's white hair or eminence," he says. And he makes no apology for his intense competitiveness or that of his peers.

"There is always the drive to measure yourself against someone else." But he sees hypocrisy in modern America's treatment of competitiveness. "We admire people most who have been intensely competitive to get to where they are, and who now don't seem competitive.

"You have to want to be the President of the United States desperately, but you must not seem too competitive. You have to act presidential, which means not overly hungry and competitive. We want people in the most competitive positions who act like they are not competitive at all."

Spetzler has chosen his own path to the legacy. If you want to be chairman of the top neurological institute in the country, and UCSF, say, is the top, then either you have to become chairman at UCSF, or move your program shoulder to shoulder with it. He makes no bones about that aim, and his belief in his ability to make it happen is marked as a measure of his arrogance or his brilliance, depending on whom you talk to.

To many top neurosurgeons around the country, Barrow's most serious impediment to reaching the top is its lack of affiliation with a university. The BNI neurosurgeons serve as the faculty of neurosurgery at the University of Arizona, 125 miles away in Tucson. But that is not being part of a university, and Spetzler is the first to admit it—indeed, to assert it. To academic physicians, the virtue of medical school affiliation is cross-fertilization. Neurology and neurosurgery, neuroscience and molecular biology and every discipline whose power might be brought to bear, all live and work under one roof, creating synergy.

But to Spetzler, whether at San Francisco or Cleveland, the medical-school connection meant competition among specialties. In university settings, "Neurology and neurosurgery do not cooperate, they compete," he says, and not merely with each other. "Neurology is in the Department of Medicine, Neurosurgery is in the Department of Surgery, and the departments are competing with each other. Then look within surgery and what do you see: nothing but competition for operating rooms, for resources. That is no virtue."

The four state-of-the art operating rooms under Spetzler's direction at Barrow are used only for neurosurgery. Yet when it counts, he can expect the closest cooperation with the cardiac surgical team headed by Ravi Koopot and Camilla Mican, the group whose precise understanding of hypothermic arrest coupled with the neurosurgical team's understanding of its effects on the brain offer the best chance for success. At the hospitals where hypothermic arrest had gone poorly, Spetzler is convinced it was not lack of any one set of skills that caused the failure, but lack of precise coordination among all the specialties involved.

The one weakness Spetzler was willing to admit to, a weakness that indeed could keep Barrow from attaining the top among world brain institutes, was in its neurology department. He was as utterly candid about neurology's weakness as he was assertive of neurosurgery's strength. Not that he would trade his independence for a medical college that might provide such a complementary strength.

He knew, as John Green knew, that BNI could not survive competition from the other great neurosurgery programs in the West without an ambitious figure heading neurology, someone to match Spetzler's ambitions in neurosurgery. The Mayo Clinic, fabled in the public imagination, now had a clinic, a foothold, in nearby Scottsdale. Unlike some, he and Green expressed no resentment over this. You either met that competition or fell to it, and he had no intention of losing. Neurology was weak; it was rudderless; it was non-existent as an academic force. Soon that would all change, he had vowed.

Spetzler now stepped to the sink between Operating Rooms 1 and 2 and, ten minutes after scrubbing out of Jack Schulte's surgery, scrubbed in again. Nurses rounded the corner wheeling a gurney on which lay an unconscious ten-year-old boy. A black steel clamp encircled his head supported by four steel rods arising from a chest harness, the device called a halo brace. Spetzler followed them into OR 2, and as evening settled, April 26 began all over again.

three | TJ

Seven-thirty on a lovely desert spring morning and Timmy Mathias whips his motocross bike down lanes of scrub mesquite and fields awaiting cotton on his way to school, his mind racing along with a ten-year-old's thoughts. Little League is underway and he made the majors; baseball is his favorite sport and sports his favorite thing, which is partly why he likes Arizona better than New Jersey: You can play outside all year. But he had a problem on the school bus a few days ago, and to keep clear of any more hassle he is biking the four miles to Horizon School, in the Phoenix suburb of Glendale, a sunbelt collage of L.A.-style traffic, cottonfields, developments, and desert. His father agreed to let him bike to school after he promised he would stay off major thoroughfares.

TJ is a "hard charger," in the language of the auto racing he loves. He does not hang back and await opportunity. He goes for it. He is double-daring, one of those lovable risk-takers, children whose racing cars mix with stuffed toys, whose motocross bikes glide down urban streets next to semis and earth-moving trucks. He's a handful. But he is keeping his promise to his father today, riding along quiet Barbara Drive. He halts briefly at the stop sign, then digs out to cross the busy four lanes of Fifty-first Avenue.

This is one of those moments his parents will replay in their minds, rewind, and replay, compulsively and against their will, as though in one terrific replay the scene they see coming will vanish like a bad dream. Tim Mathias, Sr., will wonder why Timmy did not ride down Fifty-first Avenue to the traffic light; his mother, Kerry, will ask herself why he didn't take the school bus, just today.

At 7:35 a.m., give or take a minute, a red pickup truck heading south on Fifty-first Avenue pulls from the left lane to the right lane. The driver suddenly sees a boy on a bike, who appears to be turning circles in the street. More likely the boy has seen the truck bearing down on him and, startled, is trying to turn back. He almost makes it, he is turned around; in one of those magical replays, he would make it by a hair. But this is not a magic world. At 45 mph the truck blows the bike into a ball of twisted pipe. TJ is slammed straight on by the right fender, crashes over it, and, apparently in one last effort to ward off the truck, leaves two sets of finger streaks in the dust of the fender, front to back.

All quiet. TJ lies in a bloody heap at the curb, his right leg broken so it juts at a 45-degree angle from his body. Worse, the most severe injuries are invisible ones, previously seen only in autopsies. At the top of his spine, where tough ligaments bind the first neck vertebra to the skull, there is now a clean separation. Nothing protects his delicate spinal cord. Within his skull, a hemorrhage has begun squeezing the life from his brain stem; it would not take long.

So ends the only waking hour of April 26, for TJ Mathias. As the world within him shut down so that a month would seem a day, the world around TJ began moving at alarm-bell speed.

KERRY MATHIAS HAD CRAWLED into bed just after 6 a.m., after bicycling home nearly eight miles from her night-waitress job at Dunkin' Donuts. At about the time she headed for bed, her husband was getting up. Tim was off to his trainee job with a pest-control company; that job kept him on the road nearly twelve hours a day, killing hours in the early summery heat that had descended on the Valley of the Sun in late March this year, two months ahead of schedule. They had moved here in this kind of heat, the July before: Kerry and the two Timmys, tiny Rachel, now just three, and Bob Jackson, their friend from back home at the Jersey shore who had joined the family caravan to see if his own luck might turn in new country.

They'd all piled into the rental truck loaded with their furniture, and they'd headed West, just like people had been doing for a hundred years for the same reasons. Tim had been working as a cigarette vending-machine deliverer and mechanic, Kerry as a waitress at Dunkin' Donuts. Bob couldn't work because of an accident injury but at least had some Social Security income. They pooled their money for rent, and Bob was available to stay with the kids while Tim and Kerry worked.

This was hardly something better; they were barely hanging on. First, their car had been repossessed, leaving Tim no way to get to work. But Tim's father had just visited and bought them a replacement; it was old and no beauty, but it was transportation and they were grateful for that. They would hang on and things would get better. Kerry was a firm believer that you took life one day at a time, step by step.

This morning, since she was on the night shift, Bob Jackson would see TJ off; by leaving home just before 7:30 he could get breakfast at school. The phone rang around eight, and she was initially confused with sleep. Someone from Horizon School was asking if Timmy was home sick; he had been sent home with a slight fever the day before. She was pretty sure not but checked with Bob. No, Bob said he'd gone to school. What was he wearing? There had been a bad accident; they were checking absences at area schools, and Timmy was not there yet. She looked out back: His bike was gone. Originally blue, it was a birthday present in '85 for her Thanksgiving boy – born Thanksgiving Day, 1978. She and TJ had painted the bike black just before they left New Jersey. She asked Bob what Timmy had been wearing and dutifully reported everything. And then her mind went blank. For the next forty-five minutes, if she had any thoughts, she would never remember them.

As soon as the police car pulled up, she knew. "I just grabbed Rachel and ran into the police car. I should've left her with Bobby, but who was thinking straight?" And who could have thought that the harsh weeks before would soon be the good old days. Or that she, who prided herself on being tough and no weeper, would spend a lot of the next twenty-four hours crying. She had no idea where the police car was taking her, other than to her son.

TOM SHANNON AND EARL JOHNSON would have passed each other on Fifty-first Avenue but for the traffic snarl, typical of the pre-8 a.m. rush hour. On his day off, Shannon was taking his little girls—five and one—to the medical clinic for shots, and you had to get there half an hour early or wait half the day to get in. He was southbound on Fifty-first Avenue, in the left lane; traffic ahead was stopped, but the right lane was clear, so he pulled out into the right lane, but he never did get up to speed.

Ahead was a scene he recognized too well. A crumpled bicycle, barely recognizable as such, and perhaps twelve feet beyond, a small bloody figure crumpled up against the curb. A policeman bent over the figure; a few bystanders looked on. He pulled his car diagonally to block the right lane, told his daughters to sit tight, and took off running. As he did so, he saw Earl Johnson at the same dead run, coming from across Fifty-first Avenue.

In the usual, unfortunate way of circumstance, these two who would first touch such a victim would be compassionate but ignorant strangers. Seeing the pitiable figure, the broken right thigh, the bleeding cuts up and down, one of them would scoop him into his arms to get him off the street. And would kill him in that instant. This time, both men were paramedics who lived just a few blocks from this spot. It was TJ's first lucky break.

Johnson, heading north on Fifty-first Avenue on his way to work at his Glendale fire station, got to Timmy first: "In almost any traffic accident you have to expect a neck injury, but when a bicycle is involved, it's just instinctive: You have to protect the cervical spine. First, of course, is the airway. The airway has to be open."

The cervical spine—comprising the vertebrae of the neck—begins with C1, the circular bone fused to the skull base, through the center of which the soft neural tissue of the spinal cord flows. Parallel to the spine and just in front of it runs the air pipe. When the neck is broken, the airway is frequently shut off as well. Without air, brain death occurs within minutes.

At seven thirty-seven Glendale police officer Mike Michelson had called in the accident. This was barely two minutes later.

Tom Shannon told Johnson the boy's airway was only partially open, his pulse strong but rapid. But almost immediately the boy went into a kind of rhythmic, corkscrewing contortion of his hands and arms known as decerebrate posturing. It is a major sign of severe brain injury. There was nothing they could do about that; they had to move the boy, to clear his airway. While Johnson held the boy's head and neck, slowly and carefully he and Shannon unfolded his upper body, which had been twisted to the left, so he lay flat on his back. "Call it a premonition," Johnson recalls, "but as I held his head and neck, it just didn't feel right. Usually you'd feel a strong connection, rigid muscle with a certain tone. But there was nothing."

And there was nothing more they could do. "When it's just you there, you have only your head and your hands. Your head's racing a million miles an hour, but there's nothing your hands can do."

Until you hear a blessedly familiar, shrill keening. Johnson looked up to see the yellow fire truck with its candy-apple flashing lights rushing down Fifty-first Avenue toward them. Paramedic Engine Company 54, his own unit, with Captain Steve Smith in command, had arrived with all its medical gear. It was seven forty-two, five minutes after dispatch.

Captain Smith had the Southwest ambulance crew on the scene as well as his own crew. They, Johnson and Shannon were getting IVs working, getting the boy stripped and into a Mast Suit, a jumpsuit that can be inflated to stabilize blood pressure in shock victims, getting him into a neck collar.

Paramedic's report, always staccato:

Name: unknown. Age: 10?

Pupils: Equal and reactive [to light. A good sign.]

0743: Oxygen mask.

Smith is worried about sending the boy off in the ambulance in rush hour traffic, although the crew is doing a commendable job now. He calls for the air-evac chopper.

0745: Mast Suit

0749, 0753: Blood lines in. "He had a 'hot belly'—rigid, an indicator of internal bleeding."

0755, Shannon guides in Tim Schneider's air-evac helicopter while

Johnson remains with the boy.

0757: Air evac leaves. Over the sixteen-mile flight to the St. Joseph's helipad in downtown Phoenix, flight nurse Art Russ and paramedic Neil Ashton monitor TJ's fluctuating condition.

0758: Patch. Smith was on the air to St. Joe's.

0801: "Johnny Doe" is picked up on the emergency room records of St. Joseph's Hospital and Medical Center and its associated Barrow Neurological Institute.

CHIEF RESIDENT TOM GRAHM'S Wednesday schedule was about to be canceled as he snuggled down off the men's dressing room, trying to catch forty winks. The beeper on his pager blew. By the time he reached the trauma room, junior resident Brian Fitzpatrick had begun checking the boy's cervical spine for injury. Grahm decided to stay until the first scans came in, because it would not be certain that there was neurological damage until confirmed by x-ray.

Dr. William Schiller and his trauma team were examining the boy, monitoring vital signs and preparing for the x-rays, beginning with the cervical spine. His injuries appeared devastating. Bloodied from head to toe, he had several abdominal lacerations that could have been deep enough to penetrate the intestinal wall. He had a compound fracture of the right leg. But neurologically he initially appeared uninjured. Both pupils reacted to light, both sides of his body moved in response to pain, and he was moaning. The decerebrate posturing noted in the accident report had ceased.

Suddenly the boy lashed out with his arms and cried. Now he began thrashing. Alarmed, the trauma team rushed to hold him still. He was sure to kill or paralyze himself if he had neck injuries. Schiller and Grahm decided to paralyze him with drugs; that would keep him still for now, and it appeared certain Schiller would have to undertake exploratory general surgery to confirm the extent of internal injuries, and general anesthesia would keep him still from that point onward.

Nurses Leslie Mast, Lynne Maiwurm and Sue McCoy divided up the vital duties while x-rays were shot: Hook up the respirator; he wouldn't be able to breathe while paralyzed; keep eyes on the monitors, especially noting changes in heartbeat or blood pressure that might signal crisis; keep the IV lines going; insert catheter. Then something frightening. The boy went into total paralysis, on his own. That implied damage to the brain stem. No part of the brain is as vital to the continuance of life as the stem of the brain. No brain injury could kill as quickly or, if not killing, leave the victim completely devastated. Then he came out of it, seemed to waver between neurological normalcy and paralysis on his right side.

X-rays hinted at damage to internal organs and showed internal bleeding. And there was a line of separation of the first vertebra from the skull. But x-rays would never show what was happening to the brain or portray details of the internal organs. They showed bone most clearly, missed nearly all the soft, shadowless tissues that constituted most of the brain. X-rays sometimes even miss neck fractures when they involve cartilage and ligaments rather than more-solid bone.

With respirator and lines in tow, Maiwurm took charge of the gurney and led the way to the CT scanner. This giant, enameled-steel doughnut is an x-ray machine that shoots in a complete circle, with the patient lying in the hole of the doughnut. A computer compares subtle differences in the x-ray patterns and composes detailed images of the inner body. Within the glass-enclosed control room, the medical team watched as pictures of the computer-assembed body were displayed on the monitor, in slices, head to toe.

The CT scans told Schiller all he needed to begin exploratory abdominal surgery just after 9 a.m. on Timothy I. Mathias, Jr. Now Johnny Doe had a name, and a terrified mother in the waiting room. Timmy had a ruptured spleen and damage to his liver and one kidney. Only a few years ago, these injuries would probably have proven fatal. Now, with tremendous strides in caring for trauma victims from accident site to surgery, Schiller could be hopeful, although he emphasized that the injuries were serious. He told Kerry he would have to remove Timmy's spleen but believed the bleeding could be stopped and his other organs saved. In fact, Schiller would save half his spleen, though soon that would seem a hollow victory.

KERRY NEVER EVEN SAW HIM. A doctor explained that they needed to begin exploratory surgery on TJ, and why. It was serious. She held Rachel in her arms; she couldn't let Rachel see him like this, so she couldn't go and see him herself. Now she agonized over that decision, but she couldn't let herself think why not seeing him then might turn out to be so important.

Tim was out in his truck, a few miles from the yard. He had just finished pesticide spraying on one job and would head to his next in a few minutes; then a call came to return to the office. The dispatcher's voice sounded ominous, and he wondered if he were about to be laid off. At the office his boss, Robert Ramsey, told him, "Your little boy has been in an accident. He's at St. Joseph's."

"I didn't even know where St. Joseph's was. I was kind of in a daze." Ramsey drove him downtown. It took a while to find Kerry, weary already, clutching Rachel. The little girl is at the age when her voice is fully articulate but still has the quality of a baby voice, so every word seems precocious. "The doctors are fixing TJ," she said. In the long morning's wait, it dawned on Tim that with this crisis at hand—and how bad it was he had no idea—the family had no car to get to and from the hospital. He had not completed emissions testing and paperwork needed to register their car. But everything seemed under control here. He told Kerry he would take care of that problem, then come back.

He had just gotten home, the car still unregistered, when Kerry called. Now she was tearful, and that was not like her at all. "You have to get back here quick," she said. "They're saying he might die."

Still she couldn't let herself think ahead to why not going to see him before surgery might turn out to be important. That now she might never see him alive again was not thinkable. She didn't want to explain over the phone all that the pediatric neurosurgeon had told her, or how very strong the "might die" had been. Tim drove back to St. Joe's, sure at every turn he would be stopped for driving the car unregistered. When he got there, he and Kerry were told they should not leave the hospital. Timmy's brain was bleeding, and the doctors weren't sure what, if anything, they could do.

GRAHM RAN A SET OF CT SCANS up to Spetzler as Jack Schulte's standstill began. Fitzpatrick, left to accompany Timmy into general surgery, ruminated over the remaining set of images. The scans offered little but maddening hints. Was that a shadow along the brain stem? Seemed to be. Was the shadow a hemorrhage? The brain stem did appear to be shoved back. If a hemorrhage, was it still bleeding? Just as Schiller had needed the CT scan for a detailed picture of the intestinal cavity, the neurosurgeons needed a Magnetic Resonance Imaging scan. CTs had revolutionized neurology on their introduction in the mid-seventies, for they offered finer pictures of bone, tumors and the more solid structures of the brain than had ever been available. But they were still images built up from x-rays, super-high-energy beams that pass so easily through most tissue that the delicate structures of the brain often remain transparent to them. MRI scans, to oversimplify, register tissues according to the amount of water they contain, so even the gossamer cortex of the brain shows clearly. An MRI would give a finely-discriminated picture of Timmy's brain stem, with nearly the clarity of detail seen in surgery.

But here they were stymied, and there seemed no way out. As the name implies, Magnetic Resonance Imaging uses a magnet to build its images, and the magnet is so powerful it destroys digital watches and erases credit cards. It would knock out Timmy's respirator, and that would kill him.

Without better pictures, they would have no way of knowing if something inside his head were killing him; therefore they could do nothing. There is no such thing as exploratory brain surgery. Neurosurgeons must know where they are going within an eyelash, for that is the order of magnitude of some of the brain's smallest blood vessels and nerve fibers, and as they go they must watch through the intraoperative microscope—a tool developed not quite a generation ago by Malis and Yasargil, before which this kind of surgery was virtually unthinkable.

FITZPATRICK AND STEPHEN PAPADOPOULOS, a neurosurgeon on a fellowship to refine his expertise in the spine, spent the morning and early afternoon hustling "films" up and down: to Operating Room 1, where Spetzler was in the middle of a hypothermic arrest procedure, down to the neurosurgery offices, where pediatric neurosurgeon Harold Rekate was examining young patients. Then down the hall to Volker Sonntag, Papadopoulos's mentor and Barrow's expert on the spine. X-rays, then CT scans. Then came the big break.

Barrow had just begun field testing an experimental MRI scanner, not yet in service. Its low-strength magnetic field would not interfere with respirators, but the manufacturer claimed it would produce the same fine-resolution scans as other models; it just took more time to compose its images. It had arrived only weeks earlier.

By mid-afternoon, there was a sizeable set of MRI images of Timmy Mathias's brain and spinal cord, and a critical mass of brainpower focused on them, huddled around the lighted wall panels in Barrow's patient examining area. Spetzler, Sonntag, Rekate, Fitzpatrick, Papadopoulos, an ever-shifting group of neurosurgeons looking for answers, now that the problems were coming clear. Not that clarity in this case brought joy.

"There initially didn't seem like anything we could do," Rekate said. Neuro-surgeons are not easily shocked, but that is how he describes himself as he stared at the walnut-sized blood clot pressing against the front of TJ's brain stem, finally disclosed by the new MRI. Cerebral fluid was now building up throughout the brain, and they would need to drain it to prevent massive damage—but the damage had probably already occurred.

The major shock was that the skull had been broken loose from the neck. It took a while for that to sink in. And this was no hairline fracture; the separation of the first cervical vertebra from the skull was more complete than any of them had ever seen.

Nothing held the boy's head on but his spinal cord, a few muscles, and skin. The spinal cord, to a neuro-physician, is simply brain, spidery filaments of brain running up and down the spine and to the limbs and internal organs, carrying messages in through the brain stem, commands out, gray matter and white matter just like the major volume of the brain itself. Only muscles and skin prevented TJ's spinal cord from being pulled to tatters.

How would they drain the hemorrhage? How would they reattach the skull? The usual approach for such a bleed would be through the mouth, because the brain stem lies directly behind it. But when the neurosurgeon passes through the back of the mouth, he arrives at the same tough meninges that cover and protect the brain everywhere. The hemorrhage indicated that the meninges may have ruptured; now if they cut through the mouth to drain the clot, they would infect the brain with all the microbes in the boy's mouth. The mouth and intestines can handle the rough traffic of life; the brain cannot. The clot would kill him in hours; infection would kill him in days.

The inaccessibility of the front of the brain stem was what led Spetzler to use the standstill procedure in operating on Jack Schulte. It was no small irony that here, coming through the emergency room, was an equally serious injury in the same dangerous region.

The articulated traits of personality and intelligence arise in the thick forests of connections in the cerebral cortex, and many of the finely coordinated, dazzling muscular controls of great athletes or musicians emerge in the cerebellum at the rear and beneath the cerebrum; the brain stem is life itself— breathing, heartbeat, and that most essential aspect of meaningful life, consciousness. Not pain and joy and love, but awareness arises in the brain stem.

Only a few months earlier, Spetzler had operated on a woman with a brain-stem tumor, a hellishly difficult procedure because of the need to remove tumorous tissue without damaging the healthy tissue. All had gone precisely as planned. *You couldn't have asked for a better outcome, surgically speaking.* A terrible irony. After initially appearing to recover, the woman lapsed into a coma. And she emerged from the coma into the awful state called "locked in." She was there, awake and alert, but utterly paralyzed and without sensation, able to signal only with her eyelids. It still was unclear what had gone wrong, but Spetzler was sure that a tiny perforator artery to the brain stem had ruptured or been damaged, possibly by vasospasm. The spasming of blood vessels was one of the major deadly complications of any brain surgery.

Spetzler broke the intense silence of the huddle. He suggested an approach he had developed to reach aneurysms at the front of the brain stem. Several of Spetzler's contributions to neurosurgery had come through novel approaches to impossible-to-reach areas, and he had used this unusual approach successfully. He would come in from the rear of the neck and work his way carefully around to the front of the brain stem.

Now Sonntag jumped in. He had invented a V-shaped bolt for patients with a type of arthritis that caused degeneration of the first vertebra. The bolt was used to strengthen the connection between the skull and C1. It had never been used as the sole link between skull and spine; perhaps it was worth a try.

But wasn't this all wishful thinking? Timmy now looked dead. He was not breathing on his own and not moving at all. The hemorrhage would by now be hours old, and these bleeds often killed within minutes.

"There is nothing to lose," Spetzler finally said. "If we do nothing, he will die for a certainty. If we do this, he probably will die. If we do these very difficult things, we're going to lose most of the time. But if we don't do them, we'll lose all the time."

Sonntag recalled, "From the moment he thought of his approach, as impossible as all this sounded, I knew we were going to do it."

Impossible because this was neurosurgery without rehearsal, without choreography, without precedent, and complex beyond what anyone would attempt without prior reported cases to follow as guides.

Rekate remembered, "Here we were about to start on a daunting, complex procedure that had never been tried before, going to do it now, and Spetzler was very calm about it." Neurosurgery is certainty. The neurosurgeon is confident and fears nothing. Because deep down the neurosurgeon fears only the form in which death usually pops up: Surprise! "There's nothing to lose!" Rekate said. "Imagine. There was everything to lose and every likelihood we were going to lose it."

But for Spetzler this was a defining moment of his vision of Barrow. The complete neurological institute was built by tackling any elective case with consummate skill. These are the rehearsed procedures that help neurosurgery advance incrementally, each victory the product of three interwoven factors: the surgeons' skill, the perfect cooperation of the entire medical team, and new technology. "You always trained to be your best," he says. "It's the technological advances that permit your best to be far ahead of what had been possible."

But the measure of how far you had come was here—the emergency case that in the heartbeat before now would have been a fatality, brought by the advances in emergency medicine into your hands in that broadened state of near-death. What were the respirator and the pressure suit worth? What was the value of the sophisticated training of paramedics? It stretched the fine line of death into a broad blur, and that blur could now be called opportunity.

At 2 p.m. Rekate told Kerry Mathias the grim odds. He believed there was one chance in twenty the neurosurgical team could save Timmy's life. Not that he would recover or even regain consciousness, Rekate warned, only that he would live.

"Do whatever you can," she said.

Rekate wonders in such moments what "informed consent" really means. "Patients, or those responsible for them, don't really hear the negatives; they can't. They trust you to be right. In this case, we knew we were right. I didn't see how we were going to save him, but by that time, there wasn't any doubt about his chances otherwise. Each time we looked at a new film, we were shocked all over again."

The team sent spine fellow Papadopoulos to do an on-line computer search through medical journals, through the history of such traumas as recorded in case reports, hunting for any slim comfort, any precedent that would offer hope. He found none.

Even as Spetzler judged there was nothing to lose, Rekate feared what there was to lose: Timmy, who might survive on a respirator, in a chronic vegetative state.

And then what? Kerry did not let herself think of "then what's." "One day at a time," she said.

TJ had been in a soft collar and strapped to a backboard, a position not nearly stable enough to hold his neck in surgery. The surgeons ordered a halo brace that would immobilize him as much as possible, and the orthopedics department had to cut one down to size. That meant more delay.

It was now after 6 p.m. Tom Grahm had just finished inserting the tube into the top of TJ's skull that would relieve pressure if fluid built up. He was in the halo—which resembles nothing more than a medieval torture device. A lambswool-lined jacket is fitted tightly around the chest. From it emerge four black-steel rods, running upward and inserting into clamps in the black-steel halo, which holds the head utterly rigid with a series of screws that bore through the scalp and into the skull bone. Not until the halo was in place could they roll TJ onto his stomach. Neuroanesthesiologist Steve Shedd, fresh from Jack Schulte's surgery, administered the intravenous painkillers and inhalation anesthetic, and they set to work.

Rekate, assisted by Grahm, cut down to the spinal cord, exposing the spinal processes that rise as long, sharp spikes straight out from the vertebrae. To these spikes are attached the powerful muscles of the back and those that hold the head up. It is always a bit of a shock to see the processes emerge in surgery; they give the human the look of having a dorsal fin, the spikes rising a good four to five inches out of the spine. But it takes a lot of power to hold the head up. An adult's head weighs between twenty and thirty pounds and, wagging at the end of the neck, all the leverage works against the muscles that must control it.

Rekate and Grahm step back and Spetzler steps in, prying around to the front of the spinal cord; now, on the intraoperative monitor, they can see the clot. Blood oozes, but it is dark and congealed.

"I don't know how we're going to stop that bleeding," Spetzler says, a measured, disembodied voice ever calm through any crisis. Sonntag watches the monitor, waiting. "If he dies, it will be his brain injuries that kill him," Sonntag says, brow wrinkled. "And I don't see how they can not. I just don't believe anyone has ever survived such trauma to the brain stem." He will prove correct. No one ever had.

What they fear most is an upwelling of bright, new blood, a hemorrhage that might have been held back so far by the pressure of the clot enclosed within the brain's membranes. Martin Nunemacher, the EEG technician who is monitoring Timmy's vital signs, points out that blood is a tremendous irritant to the brain, which depends on its oxygen. The neurons normally are protected by other brain cells and by an array of fibers and membranes from the caustic, alkaline blood. Only oxygen, water, nutrients, and a surprisingly small number of chemicals can cross the "blood-brain barrier." Bleeding in the brain often leads to epileptic seizures—electrical storms in which neurons damaged by the blood fire out of control.

There is no new bleed.

Sonntag now uses pliers to wrench out strips of bone from TJ's hip, strips containing marrow. He needs the marrow as seed-tissue to form new bone at the juncture between the skull and the shattered C1 vertebra. As Spetzler finishes draining the clot, Sonntag takes over, beginning the arduous process of attaching his clamp. He painstakingly wires the open ends of the "V" to the cervical vertebrae below the shattered C1. Then he fastens the point to the skull with wires looped through tiny holes drilled in the bone. And finally he squeezes the living hip marrow into the fissures of C1, where if all goes well, hard as it is to believe, it will root and grow solid.

Each of the surgeons says in turn, "That's about all we can do," then explains why it all now rests within the boy, to heal or not, if able or not. But they are all still restless. It is after 9:30 p.m. Spetzler walks repeatedly to the lighted x-ray frame, lost in thought; Sonntag paces, his hands tucked under his armpits.

"That's about all we can do."

They are not satisfied, they want to do something more. But there really is nothing more. Rekate and Grahm begin the long process of closing.

It is after midnight when Rekate meets with the Mathiases, and for the first time he can be a bit optimistic. "We accomplished exactly what we set out to do," he tells them. "There's nothing we can do now but wait. The next twenty-four to forty-eight hours should tell us a lot about whether he'll recover."

WHEN KERRY AND TIM MATHIAS stepped into the darkened room of pediatrics intensive care, early on the morning of April 27, they had not seen TJ for more than a day. He lay propped nearly upright by the halo brace in the cranked-up bed. His face and mouth were bloodied and tubes were coming out of him, everywhere it seemed. His face was swollen so badly, Tim remembers, "It looked like the pins from the halo went right through his head." Then they emerged, Kerry in tears, Tim so upset he could not speak. He had wept on his brother's shoulder that afternoon, the first time in twelve years of marriage his wife had seen him cry. He was not crying now, she noticed. "He was turned to stone."

Think about this, in the profound quiet of a hospital night: Steven Papadopoulos has reviewed the medical literature. So far, there are few C1 fracture cases to "survive"—that is, to be anything other than DOA at the hospital—and these "survivors" fall into two groups. First, there are those who suffer no brain bleeding or other damage, a fraction of that already-small number of survivors, but most of these recovered if the fracture could be mended, and not one of them had had the complete cleavage TJ had suffered. And then there are those who suffer brain injury, to any degree, of any kind. The latter all died, or worse: They became respirator-dependents. Vegetables. All dead or worse.

The hands of April 26 had done a remarkable job, woven a breathtakingly meshed tapestry. But there needed to be something more than hands at work now. Maybe it would just depend on an innate physical strength of the boy in the halo, an inborn ability to come back from the edge; maybe feelings were needed, transmitted through hands and gentle voices, an assurance that Mom and Dad were there and that other people cared about and loved him. Maybe all of the above or something still not mentioned were needed. But at the moment, the boy was still a statistic. He breathed, his heart beat, not by will but by respirator. Was he in there?

Family album. Here is the baby book of Timothy I. Mathias Jr. While he is still a toddler, his mother begins calling him "TJ"—for Tim Junior. "He walked when he was nine months old," Kerry says. "He stood up at seven months, and almost as soon as he walked he was climbing stairs and climbing out of his crib. TJ always did everything fast." Agile and strong, he still had early health problems, with allergies to citrus and dairy products. "He was in the hospital a lot," she recalls. "We'd spend a lot of time at the shore then, because the air was clean and he could play in the sand. But even when he was in the hospital, one year old, they had to put the IVs in his scalp—he'd yank them out of his arms." By age five, the allergies had disappeared.

And there is the blue bike with its beaming owner.

"Off to school again!" Kerry has written under an image of a shorter version of TJ in a red backpack, ready for second grade. He doesn't look much different in the current photos, just taller. Christmas '86: Transformers electric racing car set with proud proprietor.

Here in earlier pages are Tim, leaning up against his car, his hair dark brown. Now, at twenty-eight, it is prematurely grayed. And Kerry, smiling up from the kitchen table, looking much the same as she does today, with honey blond hair. "That was actually the night we met," she says. And he comes back with a response few husbands can match: "April 9, 1977." At his father's house in Bradley Beach, New Jersey. Both Kerry and Tim come from large families, extended by remarriages on both sides. Tim's stepmother considered Kerry's mother like family. Tim's own parents had divorced and remarried, and he was visiting his father's house that evening, as Kerry was. Timothy I. Mathias— he has no middle name; his initials spell T. I. M—was a junior at Point Pleasant High School. Kerry Konner was in the same year at Asbury Park high. Both would graduate a year later.

Tim had been raised in Phoenix until he was seven, then returned to New Jersey with his mother. Two of Tim's brothers already lived in Phoenix. In the summer of '88, when the Mathiases got to California, their original destination, they found the prices staggering. Tim suggested returning to Phoenix until they built up a nest egg. Bob Jackson, with full gray beard and long hair, looks like an adventurer, and he had been more than happy to go along on the journey. Injured in an auto accident years earlier, he could no longer follow his trade in heavy construction. The dry heat of Phoenix would be a tonic for his leg, which carries two pins from the accident. But the jobs were no better here than California, and not as good as in New Jersey.

It was just supposed to be a temporary setback.

"TJ, Mommy is here. Daddy is here. Rachel is outside with Bobby. Everything is going to be fine. You're going to get well. Your Uncle Ernie and all your cousins are outside. Your Aunt Diana is outside. Can you hear me? You're in the hospital, but everything is ok now, darlin'."

In 4 ICU, the intensive care unit where virtually all neurosurgery patients spend their first nights, sometimes all their remaining nights, Jack Schulte lies in a deep barbiturate coma. Down here two floors, in Peds ICU—the pediatric intensive care unit—Timmy Mathias lies in deep coma from which it seems impossible he will ever emerge.

A gurney moves on squeaky wheels down the dark corridor. Wheels and more wheels; the hospital moves on wheels. Gurneys, elevator wheels grinding, wheelchairs, beds, fluid stands wheeling behind, helicopter rotors, ambulances. So night circles and climbs into morning, one day higher on the calendar, Thursday, April 27.

four

A Touch of Steel

HOW DID WE END UP HERE, talking world-class neurosurgery and highest-tech science in the middle of the Sonoran Desert? Phoenix itself lacks resolution, a major metropolitan area of nearly 3 million people who drove in from the East or Midwest, or headed back from bad luck in California, a place that seems without character or history before the World Wars, a blur in time and space. But sometimes order and pattern lurk behind the blur, within chaos, and that is true resolution of one kind.

Through this lens, the bubble of a helicopter heading from the snarled traffic of Glendale eastward into downtown Phoenix, you take in the whole hollow between the cactus-dotted ridge of South Mountain on your right and the pencil-sharp tip of Squaw Peak and Camelback on your left. Back westward the boundary is wherever the sprawl stops today, flat as far as the eye can see. Ahead in the east the towering peaks of the Matzatzals and sheer cliffs of the Superstition Mountains rise, ghostly as the name, to form a basin rim beyond the spread of Scottsdale, Tempe, and Mesa.

This is the geologist's basin and range province, where volcanic mountains are thrown upward at any odd angle and the basins are what's left below, so this should properly be called the Salt River Basin, but Easterners misidentified it as the true valley of the Salt River that courses through the southern part of the city. No matter, a latter-day promoter tacked "Valley of the Sun" on the booming metro area; the Valley is what everyone calls it.

One artifact sets Phoenix apart from other cities in the desert Southwest, of human origin but so intimately bonded to the land that it seems the perfect fusion of native terrain and human will. Just as Eastern cities identify with the railroads that linked and developed them, the Valley is threaded by canals. The Highline and Western, Mormonier, San Francisco north and south, the Roosevelt, Tempe, Crosscut, and Consolidated, Grand, and Arizona. All in concrete channels, the canals permeate the Valley, watering the cotton and citrus that are now vestigal in the urban sprawl; the canals were the true vascular system of the city's birth—and re-birth.

About 700 A.D. a highly civilized people migrated from the south into this river-crossed desert basin. They brought and developed a culture surpassed in the Western Hemisphere only by those of the Incas and Mayas, but unlike those cultures, these people had no written language. Even their name is entirely a mystery, and no word of their language survives, though it must have been rich and complex. By 900 they had created a network of cities and villages with a population as high as 100,000, each interlaced with a system of canals that is a marvel to modern engineers. Experts say the canals, the most extensive in the world at that time outside Europe, could not have been aimed and leveled so true without sophisticated surveying equipment. Such tools would presuppose advanced communication and knowledge of mathematics.

They grew cotton and barley, but most significantly they displayed the true signs of civilized culture; they had leisure time and used it to pursue the arts and sports. They left behind jewelry made using the lost-wax process and they etched sea shells using acidic cactus juice. They brought to its northernmost reach a game played with a rubber ball that had to be thrown or kicked through an elevated hoop, a game played in sunken stadiums so that, unlike most Indian games, it was primarily a spectator sport.

Around 1400, they disappeared without a trace, for reasons unknown. Their historic name, Hohokam, is the word of the later Pimas for "vanished people." Many suspect that a long drought turned their canals, the lifelines of their civilization, to dust. But many civilizations have come and gone in history. Something is more haunting about these nameless Hohokam; for want of a written language, all that they were is gone as though they never existed, their entire legacy a network of lines etched with utmost precision in the desert tuff.

Nearly 500 years later along came Jack Swilling, a thirty-seven-year-old ex-Confederate officer, Indian fighter, adventurer, and hellion. Swilling came into central Arizona as a member of the party that discovered gold in the central mountains. His skull had been fractured by a gun barrel somewhere between the Mexican War and the Arizona gold camps and he carried a bullet in his left side. He took morphine and whiskey for the pain, and perhaps from a combination of those and his old head injury, sometimes he got a little crazy.

But he wasn't entirely out of his mind. While everyone else charged off after the gold, Swilling's eye caught the old Hohokam canals, and he dreamed of rebuilding an agrarian civilization. He formed a company that cleaned out the first major channel, and by March 1868, thanks to Swilling's Ditch, the first wheat and barley crops were brought in.

In October of 1870, a committee representing the farming community's population of 225 met to pick a townsite and a name. The site selected was not favored by Swilling, who fired a round of birdshot at the committee, striking one of its members. On to the name. Initially Swilling had wanted Jacksonville, after his hero Stonewall. But his sometime-sidekick, an equally wild English-man who claimed to be nobility, Daryl Duppa, put a bug in Swilling's ear. Phoenix, Lord Duppa said. Swilling reportedly dug up a Webster's dictionary right in the middle of the town meeting and found this:

In greek mythology, a bird who flew to the Egyptian city sacred to the sun god. On the altar the bird built a nest from the twigs of spice trees, then set it on fire and was consumed by the flames. When all that remained was ashes, the bird arose from its funeral pyre, reborn.

Just so, not-so-crazy Jack Swilling said. And just so the essence of the city was formulated, the quest for water as consuming a passion as the prospectors' was for gold.

It is part of gold's mystique here that people have always been even more interested in finding lost mines of it than in discovering a vein of their own. Legend has it that a Spanish family named Peralta was massacred by Apaches while trying to get its gold out of the Superstitions. An old German named Jacob Waltz claimed he had found the mine and sported nuggets around Phoenix as proof. He died before anyone proved him a seer or fool, but hardly a resident or transient in the Valley hasn't wondered if he or she might find Waltz's Lost Dutchman mine, a legend within a legend and a true part of Phoenix's fabric.

In 1949, an old prospector named James Kidd disappeared while searching for the Lost Dutchman gold mine in the Superstition Mountains, twenty miles east of Phoenix, by then a city booming with agribusiness, mining, and aviation.

Seven years later, the Arizona Estate Tax Commissioner began sifting through Kidd's safe deposit box in search of any possible legacy the miner may have left. She was startled to find that, unlike most of the old miners tracing all the way back to Jack Swilling, Kidd had hedged his bets. In addition to leaving papers for his two gold claims out past the Supersititions—the Scorpion 1 and Scorpion 2 mines—he had invested his modest income as a copper-mine worker in the stocks of such companies as the Cow Gulch Oil Company, the White Caps Gold Mining Company, Tungsten Mines Limited, Hudson Bay Mining and Smelter, and blue-chip railroad stock.

The old man was worth more than a quarter-million dollars.

His will was scrawled on lined ledger paper, dated January 2, 1946, written just this way:

this is my first and only will .... I have no heirs and have not been married in my life and after all my funeral expenses have been paid and one hundred dollars to some preacher of the gospel to say fare well at my grave sell all my property which is all in cash and stocks ... and have this balance money go in a research or some scientific proof of a soul of the human body which leaves at death I think in time their can be a Photograph of a soul leaving the human at death, James Kidd.

The wheels of government ground slowly onward. Finally, on June 6, 1967, before Judge Robert Myers of Maricopa County Superior Court, the Great Soul Trial began. No fewer than 133 claimants sought to prove either that the human soul existed or that the work they were engaged in was bona fide research that would reveal the soul *if* it existed.

The claimants ranged from dozens of parapsychology groups, spirit mediums and a California physician studying aging, all the way up to the Arizona Board of Regents, the University of Life Church, the Parapsychology Foundation, the Psychical Research Foundation, which had been founded by William James, and last but not least the Neurological Sciences Foundation, a group created by John Green to fund research at Barrow Neurological Institute because, getting a bit ahead of the story, the Roman Catholic Sisters of Mercy could only support patient care.

The trial lasted four months. The Barrow group won.

The Neurological Sciences Foundation made its case not by proving the existence of the soul, but by proving its legitimacy in the quest: Its purpose was research rather than clinical care, and it was aligned with the Catholic nuns who believed in and upheld the immortality of the human soul.

IN 1895, THE CATHOLIC SISTERS OF MERCY founded the first hospital in Phoenix, with twelve beds, naming it after their patron, St. Joseph. Business then meant agribusiness, mining, and cattle ranching. Two world wars would bring the aviation business, but it would take some time before the health care business would shoulder its way toward the top of American industry.

Fifteen miles in from the edge of the Valley, dropping down now among the high rises but still short of the Central Avenue high-rise corridor that marks the midline of downtown, the choppers bank to curve in, like a spring coiling down. First the massive bulk of St. Joseph's Hospital and Medical Center, isolated in its old Willo neighborhood, rises fortress-like, the power of its presence deriving less from height than massiveness. It looms larger and resolves into its component parts. The main building is a six-story rectangle, built with 325 beds in 1953, its long side aligned north-south facing Thomas Road with a carved stone entry-way. This entrance lets out on a traffic turnaround from the major thoroughfare. From its front, like two arms jutting at 45-degree angles, patient wings rise up, also six stories. Behind this complex facade in this building and its additions are 626 beds of the various wards and intensive care units,laboratories, EEG, the cardiovascular and general surgical operating rooms, and on the fourth floor the two pediatric and four neurosurgical operating rooms.

Major hospitals are always a confusion of architecture, the result not of accident but of colliding visions. As John Green says, each man in charge during an addition puts his own stamp on the structure, and the result is invariably a warren. The Barrow Neurological Institute building is attached right in the joint of the main building and its outreaching left arm. Adjacent to it, on the tip of that arm, the MRI suites are mortared in. The effect is no longer of a graceful oblong with outstretched arms but rather of a block-wide and -deep mass of brick and block. Behind this complex structure are angled the ancillary building containing the emergency suite and its trauma room, larger even than the Barrow building, and again tacked onto the ancillary building, curving round behind the main structure, is an eight-story patient tower. In the center of it all is a pleasant, spacious courtyard where staff and patients eat and relax in all but the hottest periods of the year.

The private offices of nine neurosurgeons occupy the first floor of the Barrow building, adding to a difficulty in resolving this group of doctors into their dual roles here. In these first-floor offices, they are private-practice neurosurgeons, seeing patients, gathering to confer with each other as partners. Robert Spetzler is just one among the nine. Throughout the rest of the building they are the principal staff of BNI, Spetzler the director, Sonntag vice-director, and so on. Four stories overhead is 4 ICU, wedged against the operating suites as the offices are wedged against the main building.

There are hints that there is something more here than private doctors' offices. The residents' library is within this first floor suite, and the residents are employees of St. Joseph's; and up and down the walkway that separates the secretaries' modules from the neurosurgeons' paneled offices, those hurrying to appointments and conferences are dressed in scrubs as often as business suits.

Intriguingly, "Barrow Neurological Institute" has in its definition the same will-o'-the-wisp quality as "mind." BNI is real. But it has almost no employees, and its few are managerial and clerical. The neurosurgeons, neurologists, and neuroanathesiologists who compose BNI do not work for it, or for St. Joseph's Hospital. Thus, although Peter Raudzens is chief of neuroanesthesia of BNI, he receives no income from the institute, nor does he have a contract with St. Joseph's or any other entity. He and the other physicians are paid by the neurosurgery patients or their insurance companies.

BNI as an entity can be distinguished from St. Joseph's Hospital but, as one business manager put it, there is only one cash register, so it is hard to define where one entity ends and another begins. The difference that had been so plain to the knowledgeable—the carpeting and decor of the hallways—eventually was obliterated by St. Joseph CEO Joseph Silva, to underscore the unity of the two. And this, in some fashion, is the kind of complexity that underlies all giant American health institutes.

As a private physicians' group, the Barrow partnership is lucrative enough to place it near the top anywhere in the country, and similar partnerships are the norm for hospital physicians whether affiliated with universities or private teaching hospitals. In fact, the physicians who have reached the pinnacle of academic medicine, serving as the faculty of medical schools, usually are limited by law on how much they may earn in private practice beyond their academic salaries. No such constraint limits the BNI neurosurgeons. And while their private salaries are not known, it is not hard to get a grasp on the power this group practice wields in this major American medical center.

A recent study of Phoenix hospitals showed that St. Joseph's took in approximately $250 million for the year in all patient costs—that is, its revenue from both direct patient payments and all third-party reimbursements, excluding fees to physicians. Fifteen hundred physicians have privileges at St. Joseph's in specialities ranging from oncology to obstetrics to cardiology; of these about five hundred are considered active because they admit most of their patients here. The nine Barrow neurosurgeons accounted for more than $50 million of the year's $250 million.

Barrow and the partnership are John Green's legacies. Though retired as director, he kept an office lined with books and photographs in the partnership suite, maintained an active role in fund-raising, and through articles and interviews tried to impress on new generations the distance neurosurgery had covered in no time at all.

JOHN GREEN WAS THE FIRST neurosurgeon in the Southwest. That seemed too primal an achievement for a man now only in his seventies, but Phoenix was only in its seventies when he arrived after World War II, a "strange, small town" to a young Chicago neurosurgeon with a head full of jet black hair, and a head full of dreams that seemed equally strange in a dusty town caught between the days of the hellion cowpoke and the hellion jet jockey.

He is a white-haired old man in his own dry seasons now, walking with obvious uncertainty of step, his voice a bit reedy and frequently tinged with frustration when he cannot pull a name up, especially as these are names of friends and mentors on the tip of his tongue. Avuncular, kind, and generous, these qualities remaining even after the power that drove him has dimmed.

There is a concept underlying the disorderly world that is the opposite of poetic justice; instantiated when Beethoven of all people becomes prematurely deaf; instantiated when John Green, silver-tongued orator of great spontaneous, unrehearsed power, loses those very gifts to a series of small strokes. His intelligence undimmed, his good humor some deliverance, he gropes for what used to pour forth from a mind as nimble as his fingers were.

Neurosurgery *itself* is only as old as Phoenix, if you want to go back to the proper beginnings—not to the first time a skull was opened surgically, but to the time of resolution.

Just a hundred years ago, in the early eighties, Rudolph Virchow made the case that the singular basis for biological function was the cell, that no invisible "humours" flowed through the body causing illness and health, that the final seat of illness and health had to be found at the cellular level.

A century is not a long time. If you are 25 years old, four of your lifetimes and you are back with the great British surgeon Victor Horsley and Scottish William Macewan, and American Harvey Cushing is just starting out. Queen Square, the world's first neurological hospital, has been open only a few years. Great surgeons arose with the great anatomists in the 1500s. Neurologists had been at work for hundreds of years, but it was discoveries in the last half of the nineteenth century that gave birth to the specialty of neurological surgery, and it was a hard birth.

Neurosurgery was born with a bad temper, short on patience, unforgiving of error and unwilling to share any glory. That was Harvey Cushing, a genius who single-handedly wrenched the specialty out of the depths of mortalities that marked its early years. Talking of Cushing is getting ahead of the story, but he is the single, sharp focus through which everything earlier passed and from which everything following emanated.

Here is the critically important fact that made it possible, about a century ago, to begin guessing where in the brain something was going wrong—where there might be a tumor, an abscess, or the congealed blood of a hemorrhage.

"In the diagnosis of disorders in other fields, the signs and symptoms lead directly to a label," notes the three-volume tome *Stroke*. That is, the cause of a malady in most of the body gives rise to specific symptoms. *But not in the brain.* "Signs and symptoms reflect the *localization* of lesion(s) in the nervous system. When one part of the brain or spinal cord is malfunctioning, the same clinical phenomenon will be seen, whether the cause of the malfunction is a tumor or a stroke or a point epileptic discharge."

Symptoms in the brain do not tell what is wrong; they tell where to look. The history of neurosurgery is the history of cerebral localization, which is the history of reading signs and symptoms and inferring where to operate.

In 1879, William Macewan of Glasgow was asked to treat a boy who had suffered a head injury days earlier, appeared to fully recover, then began having convulsions which started in his face, moved to his right arm, then affected his right leg. Macewan knew to open the boy's skull on the left side, over the recently-discovered motor cortex located at the boundary between the parietal and frontal lobes. He found and removed a blood clot. The boy recovered completely. That was the first ever. No accident, no divine inspiration, no lucky guess. He knew where to look.

Macewan owed his success to characterizations of the motor cortex by John Hughlings Jackson, whose exhaustive studies of epilepsy patients led to the first great vision of how the brain worked.

John Green wrote in Barrow's quarterly research journal that Jackson "postulated three evolutionary levels of the sensory-motor mechanism— the lowest level being the spinal cord, medulla and brain stem, the middle level being the Rolandic level, and the highest level the prefrontal lobes. He described an evolution from automatic to purposive movements and a dissolution from purposive to automatic movement."

An evolution you can watch re-enacted every morning on rounds as the residents run through the tests of the Glasgow Coma Scale. Start from the top of the brain. "Do you know what day today is?" Good, that's factual reality. "Can you say, 'Nelson Rockefeller drives a Lincoln Continental'?" That's nonsense; does the patient laugh or smile on repeating it? If so, the highest levels are functioning. End down at the brain stem. "Patient flexes to pain; loss of gag reflex; patient extends to touch." Patient's self has faded to the lowest, automatic-response level, perhaps only temporarily.

In 1870, Eduard Hitzig and Theodor Fritsch demonstrated on dogs in the laboratory that electrical stimulation of the brain produced motor response—on the side opposite the stimulation. A key piece of the puzzle for Macewan in anticipating on which side of the brain to operate. And of course, he owed much to his mentor, Joseph Lister, who taught his residents to sterilize operating rooms.

A few years later in Italy, Francesco Durante successfully removed a brain tumor from a woman, who recovered and lived for many years before he lost track of her, and shortly afterward Rickman Godlee and Victor Horsley successfully removed a tumor as Lister sterilized everything in sight, a procedure many colleagues complained was unnecessary. The patient died a week later but the surgeons declared the procedure a success, a type of judgment call still being debated in neurosurgery. From the point of view of precedent, at least, the surgery was a landmark.

Macewan took Lister's prescription for sterilization another step. While noting that infection killed most brain-surgery patients, he also observed that others suffered from the effects of the weak carbolic acid Lister required tissues to be bathed in. So Lister's pupil began aseptic surgery: Instead of sterilizing the tissue, sterilize everything else. He was ridiculed by many of his peers for operating in a sterilized, billowing gown instead of formal dress.

But of all the factors contributing to mortality, the one that stood out was failure to correctly localize the problem. Horsley's post-operative mortality was 37 percent in cases where his localization had been faulty, 8 percent when it was correct. Horsley is considered the founder of surgical neurology, but he was primarily a neurologist performing occasional neurosurgery. One took the prospect of brain surgery then far more gravely even than today.

In general, the post-operative mortality hovered between 40 and 60 percent. Those were the odds that you would die outright, never mind your chances for recovery.

In 1910, General of the Army Leonard Wood was operated on for a brain tumor by Harvey Cushing. The surgery was performed, as neurosurgeries still are in some cases, with the patient awake. A relative enthusiastically reported Wood's comments and cheerful demeanor to relatives in the waiting room. But he constantly referred to Wood in the past tense, so certain was the family that the general was as good as dead. Wood recovered completely, as the man who operated on him fully expected and predicted.

The single figure that stands over all others in the birth of neurosurgery is Harvey Cushing, who was just in training a century ago. In many ways he was the world's first neurosurgeon, rather than a general surgeon or neurologist who performed neurosurgery. Cushing's mentor at Johns Hopkins was William Halsted, one of the nineteenth century's greatest surgeons, who told him he would starve if he tried to make brain surgery a specialty, he would have so few patients.

Cushing succeeded by lowering his own operative mortality rate to less than 10 percent. He was the first of his species: None of his mentors was a neurosurgeon, and he trained the entire generation of world-class neurosurgeons to follow.

"If you look at the names of all the prominent neurosurgeons of this century, so far," John Green said, "you'll see nearly every one of them trained with Cushing, so much so that they formed the Harvey Cushing Society in his honor," the group becoming the first neurosurgical association. Among Cushing's residents were Paul Bucy, Percival Bailey and Eric Oldberg, all Green's mentors and colleagues in Chicago.

But there is probably no figure in medicine whose brilliance is so matched by darkness. One of Cushing's most famous protégés called him a very weak individual. A book published by the Congress of Neurological Surgeons detailing the lives of the first great neurosurgeons is subtitled *Feet of Iron and Clay*, and undoubtedly it was Cushing who inspired the name, representing both sides of the heroic cast.

Cushing trained at brand-new Johns Hopkins with William Halsted, who took the chief surgeon's job when William Macewan turned it down. Halsted had come from a leading New York family and graduated from Yale. As a physician he became addicted to cocaine while experimenting with it as a local anesthetic. He overcame the habit and went on to become the lion of American medicine in the nineteenth century. Halsted brought to America Lister's antiseptic practices of sterilizing the patient and operating field, and Macewan's modification of sterlizing everything else as well.

And in turn, because Halsted's scrub nurse developed a hand rash from scrubbing with antiseptic, he had the Goodyear Company make rubber gloves for her, and they slowly caught on. Sir Geoffrey Jefferson, Cushing's biographer in *Neurosurgical Giants*, noted that during his own training in 1910, the two attending surgeons hardly ever wore gloves.

However great in influence, Halsted was a terrifying figure, the image of cold and distant politeness, and Cushing wrote in Halsted's obituary that his mentor was a bad teacher and a careful but uninteresting surgeon.

However, Jefferson said, "Halsted's peculiarities arose from his perfectionism, which is always a neurotic trend, and indicate an excessive deference to the opinion of others."

No such flaw appeared in Cushing, of whom Jefferson says, "For the opinion, good or bad, of the majority of people he cared not one jot. He was fundamentally much more sure of himself, much more convinced of his own rightness—and, be it said, he had a rare flair for correctness and a rare skill in avoiding speculations that proved to be wrong."

Interestingly, Cushing and Halsted shared one personal habit: both were heavy cigarette smokers, Halsted's fingers always remembered as nicotine-stained.

Cushing was the founding neurosurgical *personality*, appropriately coming from a line of physicians older than the United States. Born in 1869, he was the son, grandson and great grandson of medical doctors. Not tall but physically aggressive, he was captain of the Yale baseball team. And he was ambitious beyond measure.

A resident who was his junior at Harvard Medical School later recalled, "He was an extremely hard man to work with, whether one was over him or under him, as his tremendous ambition for success made it impossible for him to allow anyone else to get any credit for work done....[W]hen he wanted to be, he was one of the most charming people in the world, but working with him I found that he couldn't tolerate anyone else in the limelight."

Of the two major features of his personality, the one easiest to relate is his charisma. Whether portrayed by biographers or students, Cushing's charm and the way he could light up a room with his presence are always mentioned foremost. And unlike other legendary medical figures of the period, Cushing spent his life in the operating room. Peter Black, the latest to occupy Cushing's chair at Harvard, noted one afternoon in the founder's library that Cushing's achievements were squeezed around a full day's operating schedule. And he passed on that devotion to his students.

In 1912, Cushing became founding director of neurological surgery at Peter Bent Brigham Hospital in Boston. In his library are volumes of intra-operative notes. An excellent artist, he drew exact and detailed pictures of his major cases. Renaissance man though he was, Cushing's intense devotion to the brain shows in volume after volume of drawings of hundreds of surgeries, all accompanied by equally painstaking notes on the procedures.

There was also the ruthless Cushing, equally attested, bitterly remembered even a lifetime later.

Of all Cushing's early pupils, none was more gifted than Walter Dandy. Unlike his mentor, Dandy came from a middle-class, Middle Western family of English immigrants. His father was a locomotive engineer, and Dandy grew up in Sedalia, Missouri, a railroad town. By the time he got to medical school at Johns Hopkins, he already had one trait in common with his future mentor: "a burning desire to excel.... In anything he undertook, he had to be the best."

The so-called "Cushing-Dandy Controversy" is detailed in an early volume of *Surgical Neurology*. It is impossible to fathom but easy to highlight. The feud broke out in a place central to the founding of neurosurgery, the Hunterian Laboratory at Johns Hopkins. Cushing created the lab as a place where junior residents could perform both basic and applied research on animal models, in an attempt to understand the effects of drugs and disease on the human brain under the controls of laboratory conditions.

The Hunterian is always pointed to as one of Cushing's major contributions to neurosurgery, for bringing scientific underpinnings to the practice of brain surgery. And many say Dandy was the lab's most brilliant product, because he introduced into neurosurgery many procedures that could not have been carried out successfully without the rehearsal and experimentation that the laboratory provided. The fight started in a couple of flare-ups of temper over Dandy's successful experiments that hint at envy on Cushing's part.

Then came a classic act of malevolence. When Cushing was appointed chair of neurosurgery at Brigham, he asked Dandy to join him; Dandy was delighted and quit his job at Johns Hopkins. Suddenly in mid-move, with no warning or explanation, Cushing told Dandy he had changed his mind and was *not* taking him to Boston. The brilliant Dandy now had no way even to earn a living let alone continue his training. Halsted was gone for the summer. Dandy didn't even have a place to stay until the hospital director gave him a temporary room.

Halsted found a place for him, and Dandy went on to outshine his mentor Cushing in many ways, discovering a way to drain the ventricles, the large caverns within the brain, and temporarily replace the fluid with air. That allowed the ventricles to show up on x-rays and, more importantly, allowed many brain tumors to show on x-rays before they could be localized through symptoms. In 1918, this was one of the first real breakthroughs in localizing brain injury other than by symptom, since x-rays tend to cut transparently through brain tissue.

Dandy went on to successfully remove brain tumors from formerly inaccessible locations. He had legendary surgical skills. By contrast, Cushing was not a brilliant "operator"; he had the knowledge and the vision, but his most difficult surgical work was done by his assistant, Gilbert Horrax.

Finally, Cushing accused Dandy of overlooking his mentor's contributions in tumor surgery in a major paper that Cushing saw before publication. In the course of attacking Dandy's professional ethics, Cushing said in a personal aside to Dandy, "I think you are doing yourself a great deal of harm by the tone of some of your publications. You are an independent thinker and worker, and that is not at all a bad thing. But you must not forget your manners, and this last note [article] of yours is in extremely bad taste."

Dandy was enraged, and even Cushing's biographers have been unable to find any justification for the acid in his words and tone. Dandy went on to become, by most accounts, the second major figure among America's early neurosurgeons. The rift between the two never healed. Though they were civil and polite face to face, when Cushing's name was mentioned, Dandy would mutter, "That son-of-a-bitch."

In the 1970s a historian of medicine discovered a note that may contain the germ of Cushing's invective. Cushing wrote to Dandy, "Everyone knows that you were once a pupil of mine, and though most of them know that you have far surpassed your teacher, there are at the same time certain amenities which most of us try to observe."

Far surpassed your teacher. That from a man who could never admit anyone had ever beaten him at anything. Cushing never sent the note.

Percival Bailey, ranked with Dandy among the greats of the generation following Cushing, first classified the tumors of the brain based on the cell-type of origin, while he was Cushing's resident. If Dandy emerged from the middle class, Bailey was from a background that only reached for it. Born in the dirt-poor Little Egypt section of Illinois, Bailey was the son of an alcoholic father and a hardworking but uneducated mother. Like Dandy's, Bailey's career nearly broke down before it started under Cushing's fire.

In an astonishingly sharp article in *Neurological Surgery* entitled "Pepper Pot," the nickname Cushing earned because of his terrible temper, Bailey recounted what he thought were his last days on Cushing's staff. A wealthy young woman had just been operated on for trigeminal neuralgia— pain in the large trigeminal nerve that communicates sensation and motion between brain and face. The pain-causing part of the nerve had been cut, yet Bailey was awakened in the middle of the night and told the woman was screaming in pain. His diagnosis: She was behaving hysterically to get attention, and he told her so.

Called to Cushing's office in the morning, Bailey recounts, "He was so angry that he stuttered and developed a sort of tic of his shoulder. I burst into a laugh, a purely nervous reaction that I had not planned. He stopped short, looked at me silently for a moment, turned and went back to his office. I learned afterward that he told the family I was right....

"This experience taught me a good lesson," Bailey said, "If he found he could hurt you, he took a malicious, sadistic pleasure in watching you squirm.

On the other hand, if you stood up for your rights, he respected you."

The pettiness in some of the situations Bailey recounts is stunning—and hilarious. One day, he recalled, Cushing and his Belgian assistant, Paul Martin, were operating when a group of visiting French doctors began speaking animatedly among themselves.

"'What are they saying?' asked Dr. Cushing.

"'I won't tell you,' answered Martin.

"'What do you mean?'

"'All through this operation you've been mean to me,' explained Martin. 'Now I'm mean to you.' Martin was treated with more respect thereafter."

How, then, did this tyrant become the father of neurosurgery? When Cushing began performing brain surgery, the mortality rate was between 40 and 60 percent. Within a few years, he had lowered his own to under 10 percent; he was exacting, demanding, and brutal, but his patients lived.

Bailey went on to become the leading neurosurgeon in Chicago, where John Green came under his influence.

"Bailey was the one who got me off my duff academically," Green recalls with a smile. "He showed me there is no neurosurgery without research; he showed me how the academic, scientific understanding of the brain that comes from research is the key to neurosurgery."

Green was from the then-small town of Tacoma, Washington, had gone to a small college there, then to top-rated Northwestern Medical School. There he met Eric Oldberg and fell under his spell. "Oldberg was Cushing's last sole resident," Green said. "After that, Cushing supervised the training of lots of people, from all over the world. Oldberg asked me if I would like to become a neurosurgeon. If so, he would train me; if not, he would sponsor me wherever I wanted to go. But it hooked me. The precision of the anatomy, the intellectual puzzle of the diagnosis."

And Bailey's classification of brain tumors by cell-type of origin turned out to be the single greatest predictor of long-term survival He then moved into epilepsy treatment and was a pioneer in the use of partial temporal lobe removal. Green assisted on Bailey's first seventeen cases.

Then Bailey moved into a more controversial area of neurosurgery just introduced by the Portuguese neurosurgeon Egas Moniz and hailed as a revolutionary contribution to the cure of crippling emotional disorders: prefrontal lobotomy.

The patients Moniz cured were genuinely disabled by emotional outbursts, violent seesaws of behavior the origins of which no one understood. Moniz's solution was to cut apart the connections between the most-frontal part of the cerebral lobes, which separated them from the fibers of the deep-brain center known as the limbic system. The operation indeed cured the behavior— but usually left the patients both emotionally and intellectually retarded.

"But Bailey discovered a way to limit the lobotomy," Green said, "to sever only the lower quadrants of the lobes, which effected the cure without the side effects." Green learned this procedure from Bailey and carried it with him; epilepsy and psychosurgery were to become his special areas.

The always-controversial lobotomies gave way to what was hailed as a more humane treatment without side effects—electro-shock therapy, now condemned as barbaric.

JOHN GREEN WAS in neurosurgical training when the Navy called in 1944. He was shipped to Leyte just in time for the invasion of the Philippines. The giant hospital there eventually treated 40,000 casualties, and for those with head wounds, Green was the only neurosurgeon. Working around the clock, he drove himself to exhaustion and got strep throat. That led to rheumatic fever. He spent three months convalescing at California's Corona Naval Hospital and began noticing the first symptoms of rheumatoid arthritis.

Joyce Summers was a young nurse when she and Green met. She, too, became a naval officer in the war, then became one of Green's staff nurses after the war at the Chicago Research Institute. She was of that school of strong-willed nurses who would take orders but not the abuse that was then common, abuse that the Cushing-Halsted model of training directed downward toward those on lower rungs. "There were some of those doctors who learned all the worst from their mentors," she says. "One guy in particular, the scrub nurse warned me, if he saw a nurse bending over, he'd just hook her with his foot. I said, let him try and I'll fix him with a tenaculum.

"John Green was different. He was gentle, but he had a touch of steel about him." She noticed the worry creeping into Green's talk; the winters of Chicago were beginning to take their toll. He was a neurosurgeon, and he was getting arthritis. "I said to him one day, half-joking, 'Say, let's go to Indian country.' A few days later he said, 'Are you serious?'"

Green walked into Paul Bucy's office and looked at a map of the United States dotted with pins. Red pins showed where there were board-certified neurosurgeons; yellow pins where there were candidates. In one vast area there were no pins at all: from Los Angeles to Dallas, from Denver to Mexico City. In the middle was Phoenix.

In the census of 1870, when it first appeared, Phoenix had a population of 225—164 men and 61 women, ranging in age from twenty-one to thirty. Under "occupation," ninety-six listed farmer, and there were no doctors or lawyers. Irrigation transformed the city into an agricultural center. It became the state capital after a bloody fight in the territorial legislature that would have an impact on the future of Barrow Neurological Institute. And its centrality in the state made it the chosen site for business, mostly mining, cattle, cotton and, increasingly, citrus.

Two world wars brought aviation. Two major air bases were built on either side of the Salt River Valley, Luke and Williams, and when the Second World War ended, technology brought the final catalyst to the Sun Belt boom—air conditioning.

Not that you could see a lot of that coming in 1947. Arizona had been a state for 35 years when John and Georgia Green and Joyce Summers arrived with a shipment of surgical instruments bought in Chicago. Three weeks after Green hit town, John Eisenbeiss moved back to his home state from California, becoming Arizona's second neurosurgeon and—perhaps not-surprisingly—Green's rival for the title of first and his sometime antagonist.

Here in the middle of cow, cotton and prospector country, Green had a big dream, an outlandish dream at the time: to build a neurological institute, at first to serve the growing population of Arizona but ultimately to cover the Southwest, perhaps to become a major center specializing in Green's own areas of epilepsy and psycho-surgery. By the time he began shopping the idea around town, there were about a dozen or so neurosurgeons there, and to many of them Green's plan smacked of exclusivity and elitism. There were only three major hospitals in Phoenix then, Good Samaritan, Memorial, and St. Joseph's.

The neurosurgeons generally had privileges at all three; what would the situation be in a neurological institute? Would the idea be to freeze out all but the select few? Green insisted that was not the case, but still he had skeptics.

This was a time when Joyce Summers remembers being flown all over the northern reaches of the state to care for head injuries, their pilot "a flashy blonde, made up like a show girl. But boy, could she fly that plane." And when John, Georgia and she would drive to Tucson twice a month to handle neurosurgeries there. The idea of a neurological institute seemed as remote as Chicago.

Green had for his inspiration in this pipe-dream no less a light than Wilder Penfield, who had created the Montreal Neurological Institute on just as improbable soil and lived to see it become the greatest in the world. Penfield was a Renaissance man who wrote volumes of scientific publications as well as highly readable books on the brain, biographies, and fiction. He urged the Phoenix group on and became Green's major source of spiritual support. Penfield had begun his institute with a large infusion of cash from the Rockefeller Foundation, and at his urging Green looked for the same. For a time prospects looked terrific. Then the foundation notified him that it had changed course. The foundation would now support establishment of medical facilities only in Third World countries.

That was almost more than Green could bear, spending his life bumping over dusty roads, flying into mining camps. Once, the air conditioning at the state hospital had gone out and they had to cool the operating room to survivable temperate by setting up a fan behind a block of ice. "We are a Third World country," he lamented.

By the mid-fifties the dream was eroding. UCLA, itself an upstart medical center that didn't begin growing until after World War II, now had an epilepsy center, headed by Green's good friend Paul Crandall. It would be hard to make a case for another major epilepsy center only a day's drive away. There was no medical school in Arizona and only one university, in Tucson.

It was then that investor Charles Barrow brought his desperately ill wife to see Green. Julia Barrow had had surgery for epilepsy at the world-famous Cleveland Clinic. The cause of the seizures was a tumor, and Barrow wanted Green to operate. He did so, "de-bulking" the tumor, which was all that anyone could do. Eventually it would kill her, but Green returned her to fairly good health for several years.

Green operated in the way pioneered by Penfield. He used only a local anesthetic so that he could converse with her during surgery, to make certain he was not damaging critical speech or sensory areas. In addition, he used sensors to detect any brain wave spikes that would indicate damage to the cortex or underlying brain structures.

In 1959, Julia Barrow died of her tumor. A few months later, the first new Canadian neurological institute after Montreal opened in Toronto, and Green went to the opening. He came back re-enthused, and he was always a man who could put his enthusiasms into persuasive words. This time he didn't have to. Wouldn't it be wonderful if the people of Phoenix had access to facilities like the people of Toronto had, he began telling Barrow. "Can you do it for $500,000?" Barrow replied instantly. The death of his wife, on the heels of that of his own father, William, had left Barrow searching for some way to commemorate them.

"I couldn't believe my ears," Green recalled. "After all those years, just like that."

On Penfield's advice, Green decided to locate the institute at an existing general hospital; moreover, it would be annexed directly onto the building, to be in the ebb and flow of medical activity and hospital care. St. Joseph's emerged as the hospital of choice for the location, because it had residency programs approved in all major specialties and was the only hospital in the city to offer its services free to the poor, to Green an important sign of heart.

Barrow later upped his donation to $1 million. The Sisters of Mercy, who operated St. Joseph's and several other hospitals in the West, provided $1 million to match. But there was a catch, and the catch would later turn into an important dividend. The sisters were unable to donate money for research purposes—only for medical care and medical education. Therefore Green and Barrow created the Neurological Sciences Foundation as an arm of the institute, with its sole aim to raise research money. It was 1962, and John Green was just 47.

Time, Nov. 9, 1962

Medicine Dream Institute

The nervous system is somehow involved in so many diseases and disorders, from fleeting, no-account heacaches to crippling paralyses, that doctors are often at a loss to know what part of the patient to treat first .... Merely to diagnose many cases in which the nervous system is involved takes an almost infinite variety of sensitive electronic devices. Treatment calls for gadgetry, too, and research calls for still more.

Though all major U.S. medical centers have some facilities for treating disorders of the nervous system, until now only Columbia University and the University of Illinois have had neurological institutes where all the specialties have been unified under one roof. Last week, with the dedication of the Barrow Neurological Institute in Phoenix, the U.S. got its third such organization. *The building bulged with $100,000 worth of sophisticated electronic devices.* [Author's italics]

Deep in the Brain. With eight oscilloscopes, attached to electroencephalographs, doctors at Barrow can see brain waves the moment they are generated. X-ray pictures of the brain's arteries can be taken from both front and side at half-second intervals. To locate a defective part of the brain that is causing epileptic seizures, electrodes must sometimes be delicately inserted deep into the brain itself, so the institute has an elaborate device for placing the electrodes with three-dimensional pinpoint accuracy. For the most refined diagnosis in some patients, these electrodes will be used for stimulating parts of the brain.

Of all the institute's ultramodern equipment, Director John R. Green is proudest of the massive electron microscope. Magnifying 200,000 times, it can photograph bits of matter as small as a brain cell. "We can study changes in single cells in tumors and changes due to aging," says Dr. Green. "We see this machine as ten tons of hope."

Promise of Firsts. Because tradition holds that the best medicine and research grow around a medical school in a major university, and Arizona is one of the few states that have no medical school, Phoenix seemed an unlikely place to start a neurological institute. But to Neurosurgeon Green, 47, it seemed ridiculous to wait for one to burgeon and bloom like a century plant. He longed for a local institute to save patients from having to travel hundreds or thousands of miles.

"We're not the biggest in any sense, except perhaps in the youth of our staff, and we have no 'firsts' to talk about yet," says Dr. Green. "But we expect to have a number of firsts before too long." He well may. Britain's famed neurologist Macdonald Critchley, accustomed to working on pinched budgets, helped to dedicate the Barrow equipment and said, with understandable envy: "This is a dream institute."

Wilder Penfield was there, and Percival Bailey, Eric Oldberg and Paul Bucy; all the legends of neurological medicine were on hand for Green's great day. And there was already talk of a medical school for Arizona. That would be the final piece to the dream; where else could it be located besides Phoenix, now the largest city in the state and the site of a major airport?

Looking in on that mild, bright November day, watching the smiles, hearing the speeches, the freeze-frame offers no hint of future battles or even of serendipitous good luck. But speed up the film and all manner of oddities suddenly grow, flower, vanish.

Green and the rest of the Phoenix medical powers ended up on the losing end of the most bitter fight in Arizona since the location of the state capital— and one directly related to it. The medical school was awarded to the University of Arizona in Tucson. Phoenix by then was far larger—important for providing a patient base—had a major aviation hub—important for bringing in patients on nationwide referrals—and now had a major university, Arizona State, in the suburb of Tempe. But less than a century earlier the territorial legislature had made a deal: The state capital would go to Phoenix, and the land-grant university would go to Tucson. Tucson supporters argued that a medical school should be part of that singular university.

Volker Sonntag graduated with the medical school's inaugural class in 1968 and headed off to residency under Bennett Stein, then at Tufts, with lucky timing.

Just a few years later, the medical school was thrown into a maelstrom that attracted national media attention when the physician who headed it, Merlin K. DuVal, fired the chairman of surgery, Earle Peacock. Suits and counter-suits dragged on for more than a decade, hindering the developing reputation of the surgery department.

Although the school never had a residency program in neurosurgery, it had a neurosurgical service, as any major medical institute must. The "Peacock Affair" had hardly quieted when neurosurgery hit the front pages. Chairman Alan Fleischer was sued for divorce, in a manner usually reserved for Palm Beach divorces. Fleischer was accused by his soon-to-be-ex-wife and her fiancé of sexually abusing his daughter. This would be grist for national headlines in itself, but in addition, the fiancé was Pat Conroy, author of *The Prince of Tides*, *The Great Santini*, and other best-selling novels. Shortly thereafter Fleischer, whose surgical record up to that point had been unremarkable, became the subject of several malpractice suits and a storm of criticism from colleagues. Within months, the surgery department was without neurosurgery.

BNI was invited to fill the vacuum. So two decades after Barrow opened its doors as the only major American neurological center without university affiliation, Barrow's brain surgeons became the faculty of neurosurgery at Arizona Medical Center, and a Barrow resident began spending a six-month rotation as chief resident at University Hospital—an arrangement, however, that lasted only a couple of years until Spetzler pulled the residents back to critical duties at home.

Barrow's founding came at a fortuitous moment, for it was followed by the three great technological innovations that revolutionized neurological surgery as much as Cushing had in legitimizing it as a specialty. By the middle 1960s, the intraoperative microscope was being introduced by Leonard Malis in New York and Gazi Yasargil in Switzerland. For the first time brain surgeons could see the tiny perforator blood vessels and the root hairs of nerves branching from the major stems, and could articulate with their knives the delicate foldings of the cortex and the now-giant hills and valleys of the cerebrum, cerebellum and brain stem. A decade later, Computerized Axial Tomography was invented, and some neurologists go so far as to say that that period less than twenty years ago marks the real founding point of modern neurology. In between, a form of angiography was developed that, with the aid of a computer, allowed the skull bone to be subtracted from the x-ray image, so for the first time neurosurgeons could scan the tortuous, branching stalks of the cerebral vasculature for signs of aneurysm and malformation. To Charles Wilson, this may have been a more momentous invention than even the intraoperative scope. With the addition of Magnetic Resonance Imaging a few years later, the transformation of neurosurgery was complete.

The new technology changed BNI radically, but not in relation to its sister institutions. The technological advances launched the *neurological institute* as a place where increasingly large volumes of patients went, where stroke could be treated to minimize its disastrous effects, where arterio-vascular malformations and aneurysms of increasing complexity and depth within the brain were amenable to surgical treatment before they led to stroke, where brain tumors could be excised to improve the quality and duration of life, and where epilepsy would yield itself, in the words of Yale's director of neurosurgery, Dennis Spencer, as the first neurological disorder to be truly curable through surgery.

"The scanners changed the entire complexion of both neurology and neurosurgery," Green said. "They took some of the art out of diagnosis. But they replaced the need for art with certainty. Now, when you operate, you know precisely where the lesion is. This was the aim, all along, of cerebral localization, remember. A hundred years it took. Can you imagine what the next hundred will bring?" A smiling, reflective pause, familiar for him. "I know everyone must feel this way at my age, looking into the future, but when I see these young residents, all fired up and eager, I wish I were starting out now, with all those discoveries ahead of me that they are going to be part of."

five

Crystal Shattering

JENNIFER TURNER IS a born-again romantic. No matter how many times life shoves her down, she'll get right up again and will not give in to seeing things dismally. As she stands before the mirror combing her gorgeous long honey-blond hair, she feels terrifically pleased with herself; dressed to the hilt and sure to turn some heads. She found the prettiest blue dress, with a white bib, and blue shoes to match. This is important. When things aren't going well, you pull yourself together and put on your best face, smile and light up the room, and soon everything gets back on track. It works; it will work.

Born in Yuma in 1958, when nearly all Arizona was nothing more than desert criss-crossed with blacktop iced on hardtack. Raised in Avondale out in the cotton country west of Phoenix, flat all the way to the contrasting Estrella Mountains rising black and dusty to the south, the jets of giant Luke Air Force base roaring through the skies in a like contrast to her sleepy Western town. In Avondale, everybody knew everybody's kids and nobody locked doors. She had always loved Avondale.

Then the sixties were turning into the seventies, and along with rock 'n' roll and the national fads and styles that percolated down to every corner of the country came the drugs that did for small towns just what they did for the city neighborhoods—made the boredom go away and took the security away with it. Fueled the romantic dreams. Up up and away; in the morning sometimes left a new dullness, a new bottom a little lower than the old one, which you had to work a little harder to make go away. She never did hard drugs in high school, just smoked marijuana and drank beer. She graduated, an achievement of real pride, went on to get a waitressing job at the golf and country club a few miles away, frequented by retired folks and Air Force and civilian employees.

The waitressing job paid the bills but was no part of the dream; the dream was to get married and raise a family. She met Anthony, who was terrific. Handsome as hell, but more important than that, someone who wanted to better himself. When they met he was a dishwasher, but soon he was working in mobile home construction, a better job that had possibilities. They talked about both going back to school. She became pregnant and they got married. December 15, 1979, a beautiful day. And then in June 1980 they had a beautiful son with a beautiful name to match, Marc Anthony. Very romantic.

She applied her eye shadow now. She was always very careful, very fussy, about matching her eye shadow to her clothing, so she'd look just real nice. Dolled up. *Women really do get weird about having to look just right.* A wave passed across her. Not a pain or anything, just, like, a chill, a shadow crossing the sun for a few seconds.

That was what it was like, the bad times in her life; you could never put your finger on just what was starting to go wrong, and after it passed all you knew was it was past. After seven years, she had left Anthony. Even now she wasn't sure why; she only knew she had not seen her departure as a finality, so she was hurt, and surprised she was so hurt, when Anthony had gotten his new girlfriend pregnant. He had not wanted to have more children; that was one of the things between them. She had left him. That was her worst mistake. And he'd gotten in all kinds of trouble since. She'd had to write a letter to keep him out of jail. Then she met an Air Force master sergeant and married him, her second worst mistake. the beginning of the journey down. It had seemed like a good, solid idea. He had security, a good income and benefits; she would be able to devote more time to Marc Anthony, who was seven and just the brightest boy.

It turned out to be a short trip, but it ended a long way down. They moved to Tucson. He was an alcoholic, and she became an alcoholic. He was abusive. She didn't take it well. He threw her out. She had seventy dollars to her name and was hooked on booze and knew it. She was terrified, one step away from being homeless and here she had this beautiful son and no real job skills and seventy dollars. So she came back home to Avondale and moved in with her friend Linda and her husband and kids, all of them packed at first into a trailer big enough for one family. And she got a job. And she went to a drug rehab center. She was surprised to find she was the only one in her group there for alcohol abuse; all the other women were there for drugs. Hard drugs, soft drugs, prescription drugs, any and every drug.

She licked the alcohol.

She was working now and trying to go to school to learn data processing. She had her own trailer near Linda's. But life was very tough. She would get at most four or five hours of sleep a night. On and on with no break in sight. She allowed herself only one helper-through, and it seemed as safe and easy as any pill could be. With a few whiffs of a street amphetamine called crystal, she coped. The thing about crystal was, it didn't send you soaring only to bring you crashing down again; she'd seen plenty of people do that with cocaine, heroin, the hard stuff. Crystal just got you wide awake and kept you there, and if you didn't take it for a while, you just felt real tired.

So there she was, on the road back. In a place where dreams were possible again. She'd get home from work, take a little crystal in the evening, a little more later. And when she'd get up, like this morning, at 5:30, she'd take Marc Anthony over to Linda's, so he could have breakfast and get ready for school with Linda's kids, then go to work herself. *Another wave came, right now, like a big cloud passing over.* Suddenly she was sweltering, as though the sun emerging from behind the cloud had burned all the air out of the world. She couldn't breath and a pain coursed up her neck. She ran outside, but when she got outside it was freezing. The world was spinning out of control. The pain in her head was intense.

It's running down my neck. Oh God!

This will go away, be calm. It was scorching; now it was freezing. *This is not good. Oh man. This is not good at all. I can't see.* She is stumbling along the pathway in the freezing air.

"Sit down," Linda said.

"I need to get to a doctor," Jennifer said, and then let herself break down and cry.

Look inside her head, as will be easy in a few hours by plastering the angiogram x-rays against an illuminated screen. See where the lines of arteries around and through the brain articulate like the branching and swirling of tumbleweed stalks, growing ever finer but more dense as they split off from larger trunklines. Look at the trunklines; this is getting to be strangely familiar territory; we are like hikers believing we are marching straight through time, yet toward the end of an April that never comes.

Instead of finding the end of April we keep finding new expressions of this one theme: The left and right vertebral arteries come up the front of the spinal cord (as the carotids come up in the neck). Right at the base of the brain, the vertebrals join into the single basilar artery. The basilar runs up the brain stem, the most critical part of the brain for the simple continuance of life, sending a few smaller branch arteries off to feed that stalk of neural tissue, and then it divides into the left and right posterior cerebellar arteries that feed the cerebellum. You can see the stalk of the large basilar artery run up the brain stem, and right at that arterial "Y," where the pons bulges out over the brain stem like an Adam's apple and the artery enters the circle of Willis, the basilar balloons like a gum bubble, thinning dangerously as it swells, thinning enough for blood to perfuse the now-membranous tube and hemorrhage into the brain. It is an aneurysm, "right up against her soul," a technician later will say. Right up against the brain stem, where dwell heartbeat, breathing, wakefulness. Take them away and what have you got?

FRIDAY NIGHT CALL WAS THE WORST. Or was it Saturday? Saturday night was busier but Sunday usually was quieter than Saturday, meaning you caught it both night and day on Friday night call. Bruce Cherny had been on the run all day and now, as he tried to complete his afternoon patient rounds following Spetzler rounds. That was the thing about the Boss: Imagine sticking around till 4 or 5 o'clock on a Friday for rounds when you are the boss. True, Friday Spetzler rounds were usually earlier than the rest of the week, but that was a blessing for the residents as much as Spetzler and they wished for them all to be early.

And here is Cherny steaming down the hall in 6 East thinking he might get dinner soon and wouldn't you know? *Trauma team, to the emergency room. Trauma* heard you the first time *team to the emergency room. Trauma team* oh yeah *to the emergency room.* Down six flights two stairs at a time and just in time for the medevac chopper from Maryvale Clinic. The patient came in in a wheelchair and was conscious, but she was hysterical. He had to calm her down.

"I can't die," she said. "My little boy is staying with a friend. I can't die."

The call from Maryvale referred her to Joe Zabramski, who had joined the staff just a year ago at the end of a fellowship, that on the heels of chief residency. "Z" had interests similar to Spetzler's in specialization: vascular neurosurgery, and a terrific sense for research. And fortunately, here he was.

Zabramski came in the examining room as Cherny was trying to calm the patient. He had no better luck; she would calm down for a while and then become frightened again.

Within a short while Zabramski had seen her scans and talked to Spetzler, and he knew what had to be done. "You have an aneurysm in your brain," he said. "That's a swelling in an artery, and this is in one of the major arteries of your brain." And once having started, there was never any point in stopping, because there was certainly no turning back: "In order to get to this aneurysm, we're going to have to perform a high-risk procedure, but we've done it before very successfully. It's called hypothermic arrest."

"I don't want to die," Jennifer cried out.

"We don't want you to die," Zabramski said, finding it hard to believe that with the amount of blood he saw on her scan, from a massive hemorrhage beneath the meninges, she could be awake and alert, let alone so agitated. How do you tell a 30-year-old woman what you want her consent for? "I'm going to try very hard not to let you die. In order to get to the aneurysm, in this procedure, we will have to stop your heart for a short period of time, then we will start –"

"But I'll die if you stop my heart!" She shouted. Didn't they understand? How could she get through to them here. "I'll die!"

"Ma'am, if your aneurysm bursts before I can operate, *then you will die.* Listen to what I'm saying. And if you don't calm down, it may very well burst. If you calm down, I think I can save you. But if you don't calm down, you will die."

And she calmed down. Way down. Sunk to a miserable low that was awful to see. "You're not going to cut my hair," she said emphatically, stroking her long, blond hair. "I don't care what you do to me, but you cannot cut my hair!"

MOST OF THE NINE RESIDENTS on Saturday morning rounds wore running shoes, so they would have been a silent if rhythmically-moving procession marching down the hallway at quicktime, but someone was wearing what sounded like leather-soled shoes this morning, and that heightened the military air. Clickclick, clickclick, clickclick.

Here is Jack Schulte, 48-hours-plus post op, still deeply comatose, although they had begun weaning him from the barbiturates that had helped bring him to arrest for surgery. At his age, 64, they would need to bring him back slowly. Bringing people out of arrest slowly had turned out to be important, just as their research had shown that damage in earlier cases had been caused by re-warming the patient too quickly, setting in motion too high a demand by all those billions of brain cells for everything they needed to live.

And here is Jennifer Turner, about to take the same journey. A pretty woman, quiet, with a shy smile, small of build—just 95 pounds—with short-cropped hair. Alert, jumpy, her eyes darting at each of the residents. Soon Zabramski would shave her in a high arc over her left ear, nearly to the crown. They were setting up the OR now, and the heart bypass team was expected within the hour.

Moving down the two-bed rooms of the fourth-floor intensive care unit, every morning the residents found the complete spectrum of alertness and control, although those at the upper end of consciousness, registering 14 or 15 on the Glasgow Coma Scale, were generally headed out to "the floor" on that day, to one of the regular BNI units, unless some other test showed a fluctuation or there was infection or another complication that so far had not interfered with alertness.

What is alertness? Degree of consciousness, obviously, and we all have reasonable, intuitive ways of gauging others' alertness. Doctors have always observed very specific correlates of these degrees of consciousness, but until just over a decade ago, they had no means of quantifying their observations. Volker Sonntag, BNI's vice chairman, spine expert and head of residency, impresses new residents at their first weekly meeting with the importance of the Glasgow Coma Scale, which they soon know by heart. With it, the doctor tests a patients responses to quick tests in each of three areas, assigning specified points to each response. Then the points are totaled. The resulting numbers allow precise communication of a patient's alertness.

Sonntag had already finished his training when the GCS was introduced. Without it, "I'd call you on the phone and say, I've got a guy who's lethargic, or semi-conscious, or stuporous. And that might mean different things to each of us."

Then the scale was developed by Drs. Teasdale and Jannet of Glasgow as a barometer of consciousness.

GLASGOW COMA SCALE

EYES OPEN	Spontaneous	4
	To verbal command	3
	To pain	2
	No response	1
BEST MOTOR RESPONSE		
To verbal command	Obeys	6
To painful stimulus	Localizes pain	5
	Flexion-withdrawal	4
	Flexion-abnormal	3
	Extension	2
	No response	1
BEST VERBAL RESPONSE	Oriented and converses	5
	Disoriented and converses	4
	Inappropriate words	3
	No response	1
TOTAL		(3–15)

For example, if a patient only opens his eyes when commanded, then they drop closed again, that is a sign of diminished consciousness. If they do not open on command but do open to pain—a pinch of the skin—that marks still more-diminished consciousness. And if they do not open at all, more diminished still. Motor responses similarly show a steady depression of alertness: patients who respond to a pinch by reaching for the sore spot score a 5, those reflexively extending their limbs to a painful stimulus are at the lowest edge of coma. Thus the GCS has offered yet another way of articulating the "gray blob" that coma had represented.

Those introduced to the scale notice immediately that a dead person would register a "3" on the scale, for there are no "0" options. Naturally that's the source of considerable graveyard humor: It's a measure of the neurosurgeons' eternal optimism—Even when you're dead you score a 3; or, you get 3 points just for showing up.

But there are serious reasons for the lower limit of 3. The score is a "litmus test" of consciousness, not a test of brain death, and the number is a reminder that this is only a neurological snapshot; the patient may have excellent heartbeat and respiration, for example. Finally, the test scores presume the patient is not on barbiturates or other drugs, or quadriplegic, or in any one of several other conditions that could throw off the numbers. But when a resident notifies the attending neurosurgeon that a patient's GCS has dropped significantly, an alarm bell goes off and more discriminating tests are used. In the emergency room, the major break points are these: A score of 11 to 12 is usually the sign of a concussion; from 8 through 11 usually marks a moderate head injury, and below 8 a severe head injury.

The eyes are the key to the most serious tests of coma and brain-stem injury. The windows on the soul, of all the obvious organs to examine. "Many people say you can judge 90 percent of coma with a good eye exam," Sonntag says. Dilated pupils which do not respond to light are the mark of severe brain-stem injury. Then there is the doll's-eye reflex. If a patient's head is turned, primitive controls in the brain stem should keep the eyes steady—controls that are part of the vestibulo-ocular reflex, or VOR, one of evolution's most intriguing and oldest inventions for survival. If the eyes remain unmoving, like a doll's painted eyes, the patient is usually near death.

The VOR keeps the eyes steadily on target regardless of how we run or jump. The importance of vision to modern humans can be measured by the numbers and varieties of metaphors we use relating complex ideas to those that can be beheld visually. The importance of vision in evolution can be gleaned from the early development of sophisticated eye controls; the VOR in primitive fish is as well-developed as in humans. And the importance of vision in mammalian development is suggested by the amount of brain power devoted to it. Vision occupies the entire occipital lobe at the rear of the brain, the most protected area of the upper brain. Of the 12 cranial nerves, which mostly control sense and movement in the head and neck, one governs seeing itself—the optic nerve—and three govern eye motion.

JENNIFER TURNER'S blue eyes are closed, but no GCS evaluation will tell where she is; a series of anesthetics beginning with a soporiphic to make her drowsy and concluding now with deadening barbiturates have put her beyond such simple tests. Now only the machines of the operating room under neuroanesthesiologist Karl Hendrickson's watchful eyes can read the messages of her brain's activity, some as faint as radio messages from distant stars.

The neuron is the key to brain function. It fires or it does not, depending on the messages coming across its incoming dendrites. Some of the incoming signals are inhibitory, tending to prevent the neuron's firing; others excitatory. The incoming messages function in a simple additive fashion; if the sum of the incoming impulses, which may number in the tens of thousands, is below the neuron's firing threshold, it lies still; if above the threshold, the neuron fires, sending a single, powerful pulse of unvarying magnitude down the length of its axon. That's it.

How can you tell which messages are inhibitory and which are excitatory? Overall, researchers can't yet, but they can study these patterns of excitation and inhibition in as simple creatures as sea slugs and see the same relationships among neurons as in primates. The conclusion is surprising and inescapable: By several orders of magnitude, most of the signals a neuron gets are inhibitory.

Peter Raudzens, chief of neuroanesthesiology, explains the anomaly simply. Look at a tiger springing, the very image of coordinated grace and muscular power. To achieve this, imagine all the cells in the tiger's brain firing at once, and then inhibit out all but those that add up to that fluid motion, inhibit out all those that do not contribute to the power and synchrony. Perfectly analogous to Michelangelo's depiction of creating a sculpture: Cut away all the marble that is not part of the figure.

A neat enough picture so far, but there is an error at the heart of our metaphors of brain activity that masks the truly astonishing nature of the communication going on. The metaphors come from the world of electric circuits and, more recently and more powerfully, from the world of computers. We see the brain as a computer. A signal goes in one end of a neuron, comes out the other, affects other neurons, just like an electric pulse running through the switches of a computer chip; the "on-off" nature of the neuron's firing lends itself to the image. It is entirely wrong.

The only energy that is "incoming" to the neuron is the signal energy; each neuron's *outgoing* energy is all its own, the product of its cellular metabolism. Look at it this way. Here is a line of army recruits; we had been imagining one shoving the other, whose arm shoves the next, on down the line. Wrong. Instead, the first in line calls to the next, who turns, and calls to the next, who turns, and so on down the line. Yes, there is signalling energy expended that is the cause of the reaction, but it is not the energy of the reaction.

In the 100-billion-cell light show of the brain, then, as each neuron sends one of dozens of neurotransmitters to signal other neurons, which fire or do not fire neurotransmitter in response, is there any word in English to generalize for every case what the neurons are exchanging? Only one: information.

Now consider that there are 100 billion neurons, each firing every second or so. And consider that some neurons fire at dendrites of neurons that fire back at *their* dendrites, directly or in multi-neuron loops. Imagine trying to control traffic in such a communications network. The brain does, usually flawlessly. Many firings of many neurons are modulating signals; think of them as functioning like the orchestra's percussion section. They keep the brain operating in a harmony more magnificent and complex than any yet written. Epilepsy is the symptom of neurons firing out of control, creating an electrical storm instead of a finely modulated wave pattern, usually just in one small area but potentially spreading across the entire brain.

Look at the EEG monitor, whose electrodes dot Jennifer Turner's scalp; across the screen stream regular spikes of brainwaves, marching in groups of anywhere from 2 to 30 per second, like soldiers in file. The signals represent those modulating neurons firing in coordination, apparently setting the clocks of all the rest.

"Brain waves" tracing across a monitor are so much part of popular medical imagery that the EEG seems an ancient rather than recent invention. It was put into use just 50 years before it read Jennifer Turner's brain activity. Percival Bailey was persuaded by colleague Frederic Gibbs at Illinois to use the results of the magnificent new machine to help diagnose epilepsy.

Hans Berger of Germany had for years conducted experiments based on the fact that neurons give off electrical pulses. The electrical nature of brain communication was well-known: Stimulating the motor areas of the brain with a low-voltage electrical pulse would produce motion in the corresponding limb; stimulating a sensory region would produce sensation in the appropriate area. By the late 1930s, Wilder Penfield was already using such stimulation intraoperatively to locate important motor, sensory and speech areas during surgery for epilepsy at the Montreal Neurological Institute.

But measuring brainwaves was much harder than stimulating neurons, because nearly all of what a scalp electrode picks up is the noise from most of the 100 billion cells carrying out individual activity. Berger had to find a way to subtract out this noise and magnify the aligned signals. He finally produced a machine that was barely able to measure these currents traveling without opening the skull, and he is credited with inventing the EEG. But he was declared a political undesirable by the Nazis and was forced to stop his research, before his laboratory creation could be turned into a medical instrument.

Gibbs had visited Berger. He persuaded a Boston engineer named John Grass to attempt to build the machine, and build it as a reliable clinical instrument. Grass was at work on the precursor technology to radar, trying to develop sensors that would pick up faint returning radio waves and map them. The problems were surprisingly similar. Whether you were trying to bounce a radio wave off a distant aircraft and read the return signal or to read the spontaneous pulse of microscopic brain cells, the major hurdle was to subtract noise and amplify the desired signal. Grass succeeded. The Grass

Instrument Company in suburban Boston, which he operates with his wife, Ellen, is still a major manufacturer of the EEG. Ellen Grass, a biologist, is a frequent lecturer and presenter at medical and scientific meetings. And John Grass, a plain-spoken, unassuming engineer in plaid shirt and work slacks, still works out of the firm's institutional-green quonset building, where his first EEG occupies a drafty storeroom.

Built before the cathode ray tube made the monitor possible, Grass's first working model used the brain's amplified modulating signals to operate magnetic switches, which sent a pencil-beam of light skipping up and down a scrolling sheet of photographic paper. It had to be operated in the dark. Soon he amplified the signal enough that the switches would let a pen plotter do the skipping. Days-long EEGs on epilepsy patients still are recorded that way. When Barrow's Grass Instrument Co. machine started acting up a couple of years ago last Thanksgiving, a phone call brought John Grass to the rescue. He crawled among the hospital's impanelled cabling till he found wiring that was interfering with the machine.

The EEG measures different varieties of modulating firings, each with its own identifying frequency. The brain waves of rest, called alpha waves, emanate from the Reticular Activating System and spread upward to the parietal region under the crown; as you fall asleep, those waves move forward. And there are synchronized—S—and desynchronized—D—rhythms marking deep or lighter sleep.

The EEG signals now spiking across Jennifer Turner's green monitor carry an electrical potential of 50 to 80 microvolts. If that represents the simultaneous firing of just 10 percent of the 100 billion nerve cells, you get some idea of the incredible fineness of the brain's electrical system. (It is estimated that a plain steel door has a magnetic field a million times that of the brain.) On the other hand, if this EEG reading represents an averaging of the firing power of 10 billion cells, that offers a hint of the precise *coordination* of that system. It is as though we are flying over a meadow of ten billion fireflies and see, instead of a random patterns of sparks, a steady drumbeat of almost perfectly-coordinated flashes.

The electro-chemistry of these neural firings now is well understood. But the regular flowing of brainwaves through the universe of the cortex, and what such waves mean in particular regions at particular times, is still largely a mystery. At any given moment, throughout the vast domains of neural networks of the cerebral cortex, the billions of individual firings are composed into very regular waves, complete with cross-currents and local changes, that tell much of the "weather of consciousness." And changes in that "weather" parallel changes in the conscious state closely monitored by the neuro-anesthesiologists.

Moreover, Raudzens noted, so important is the coordination of these firings that many patients whose overall brain activity is normal show severe mental impairment and dysfunction, because the coordination of these pulses is not correct. It's as though two ocean wave currents that normally flow parallel suddenly run head to head or at some oblique angle, with a resulting fragmentation and loss of power.

And "brain weather" is even more noticeably affected in the ancient scourge of epilepsy, which is finally being understood by researchers and successfully treated in a variety of ways, including surgically, to remove the focus of storming cells.

Here in OR 1, this much is clear: Given the level and pattern of firings, Karl Hendrickson knows that this brain is not conscious; when the waves go away altogether, this brain will be indistinguishable from one that is dead, and in a few hours, when the drip of chemicals through the IV into Turner's brain is cut off, the returning pulse of brain waves will map out the return of consciousness.

"Body temperature 30." That's 86 Fahrenheit. The cardiovascular team this morning is headed by Dr. Ravi Koopot, and he had worked with quick, deft strokes to open an incision in Turner's right thigh, to place the plastic tubing into the femoral artery. Then began the bypassing of Turner's blood, although for a time, while everything was brought into sync, her heart still pumped into the femoral tube, over to the bypass machine, and back into her again. Whenever the neurosurgeons gave the word, her heart would be stopped.

Zabramski had begun operating just after 9 a.m., Spetzler joining him right after opening. Spetzler remained, carrying out some of the procedure himself, closely monitoring every dose of every drug dripped through the IV. For every new life-saving procedure there was a new threat. Indeed, that was what made hypothermic arrest so challenging. It was a complex set of carefully modulated treatments, of precisely the right drugs administered in precisely the right doses, and of similarly precise coordination among groups of people used to working fairly independently: neurosurgeons, cardiac surgeons, anesthesiologists, and all their related specialty teams from blood perfusionists to nurses.

"We've now extended the safe period for hypothermic arrest from one hour to 90 minutes in the primate," Spetzler said. "Our goal is to extend it to three hours. If we can reach that goal, there are many more procedures now undoable that will be accessible to us" because the threat of bleeding will be eliminated. But they have not tried to keep a human under that long.

Brian Fitzpatrick, the resident assisting Zabramski and Spetzler this morning, noted that some studies already had been done extending arrest in dogs for far longer. And dogs are higher mammals—usually the critical distinction in choosing a model. To say that a given mix of drugs will knock out even a mouse, a lower mammal, and return it to normal is often meaningless in trying to predict what it will do to a human.

Zabramski shot back, "But how much brain does it take for a dog to be a dog? That's the whole problem. How do you know if you've brought a dog all the way back?" And that is the whole problem of neurosurgery in a nutshell, as it will play out over the next weeks and months in an endless variety of ways: How do you know you have restored a human being to perfectly normal— same personality, same likes and dislikes, memories, hopes? And if sometimes that's hard to tell with a human being, how do you tell in an animal that cannot speak, play chess, or appreciate Mozart? The best you could do in research, which was where Zabramski was putting much of his energy in these early years, was to come up with as close-to-human a model as possible. For now, that meant the baboon.

And here's what "close as possible" often means. Recently they had clamped off a cerebral artery of a baboon for 45 minutes to induce a stroke; they then would give the ape what they hoped would be the perfect balance of experimental drugs to reverse the effects of the stroke. But after 45 minutes, the baboon's collateral blood flow—blood coming across the top of the brain from the opposite hemisphere, a safeguard system—was so strong that it never had a stroke. End of experiment. They unclamped and closed, a surgery painstaking, antiseptic and monitored—though no match for those here on the fourth floor.

Some patients, similarly, had aneurysms burst and even after hours of ischemia—interruption of blood flow—recovered 100 percent, because of strong collateral blood flow or for reasons unknown. Others lost vital brain function forever in just minutes. All their efforts, here and in research, were toward trying to find universal solutions to universal problems, then adapt them precisely to the demands of exquisitely individual brains.

Now, early afternoon already, Zabramski is nearing his destination. The entrance just behind and below the ear took him in beneath the right temporal lobe. If you hold your hand flat, then curl the fingers at the middle joint, keeping the thumb aligned straight, the thumb resembles the temporal lobe. Above, the parietal, sweeping forward to the curling fingers of the frontal lobe. The heel of the hand would be the occipital lobe, which rests atop the cerebellum that swells out behind the brain stem. To get to the basilar artery, he must cut through the tentorium, then move to the front of the brain stem. The tentorium, or "tent," is a membrane walling off the cerebellum. As he tugs back the tent, a blob of blood oozes.

"Just from the small blood vessels of the tent," Fitzpatrick observes, watching the monitor. "If that were an aneurysm bleeding, blood would fill the whole field."

Behind the tent, the third nerve emerges on its course from the brain stem to the eyes, where it will control eye motion, and there is the posterior cerebral artery, which comes off the circle of Willis just ahead of the basilar juncture, so we're getting close. The posterior cerebral will feed the cerebrum and its cortex. Next to it, the superior cerebellar artery that supplies the cerebellum with blood, and just behind them, something looms; not quite clear yet but huge.

"My God," Zabramski says. "Look at the size of that." The aneurysm emerges, a huge beehive; angry red, so thin is the wall of the basilar artery. "This is as far as we go. That thing might burst. Start bypass."

Soon Jennifer's heart stops, and the steady reading of temperatures begins. Now she is down to 77 degrees Fahrenheit, but her brain temperature still lags at 84. Spetzler calls over to Koopot, "We want her at about 18 degrees," down around 64 Fahrenheit. The temperature, like the mix of drugs, has been figured as precisely as possible based on Turner's age, weight, general health.

Spetzler and Zabramski now stand up, nod to each other, and scrub out. There will be time now to catch up on other matters while waiting for the right temperature and for the blood to drain.

Spetzler heads for his office, where he will have Saturday quiet to work for nearly an hour on a matter crucial to BNI's future.

At 1:29, the pumps are turned off. No blood flows anywhere in Jennifer's body. Blood is still draining, but the aneurysm has collapsed; there is no danger of rupture at least; the worst fear is over. Tiny perforators can be seen for the first time on this clear field, like root hairs against the ropy basilar artery.

Spetzler and Zabramski are telephoned and in minutes are scrubbing in again.

And now, to work. The aneurysm is flaccid and pale as Zabramski seats the Yasargil 9-mm clip in the special pliers that force its spring open. It is all over startlingly fast. The clip is seated over the bulbous neck of the aneurysm, so blood can still flow through the major, undamaged portion of the artery.

"Pumps on at 1:40, after 11 minutes with no flow."

"Okay, very nice," Spetzler says to Zabramski, and as always, as he scrubs out, says, "Thank you all very much." Now time would tell the outcome.

Training

S P E T Z L E R   H E A D S   F O R   H I S   O F F I C E.
It is Saturday-quiet down in the first floor annex that houses the neuro-surgical partnership, the private corporation of the nine attending neurosurgeons of Barrow Neurological Institute.

He flicked on his office TV monitor and immediately was looking down on OR 1, a fly on the wall. If the intraoperative microscope were in place, he would be looking at Jennifer Turner's aneurysm, as the neurosurgeon would be. It was easy for everyone to forget the Boss might be watching. More than once he had been called because a complication had occurred or a decision needed to be made by him, and although mere seconds had passed the caller would hear a crisp, "I was wondering when you would get around to calling me," as though they had lollygagged.

Spetzler's office was not exceptionally large, but as a refuge it was a work of art. He had replaced the long expanse of plate-glass windows facing the Third Avenue entrance to St. Joseph's and BNI with etched, frosted glass, so the large room remained airy but the light was soft. It was actually a double room, split by a bookcase divider. Seated at his desk now, microcassette recorder in hand, he faced a large tank in which tropical fish swim among colorful plants waving in an induced current. The monitor was up at the ceiling, to his right.

On the opposite side of the divider was his true escape within the BNI walls and his pride and joy: an ebony upright piano on which he can play his favorite Mozart or Beethoven. But wouldn't patients entering the neurosurgeons' offices in pain or grief find it jolting to hear the crash of a piano in fortissimo above soft office voices? They hear nothing. Although the piano was concert quality in tone, it was fully electronic, and with a flick of a switch Spetzler's music can be heard only through headphones. He was crazy about technology. But he was not here for a concerto today. He was putting the finishing touches on a matter both difficult and critical to BNI's future as America's leading neurological institute, a ranking certainly more than a pipe dream but far from universally agreed upon by the directors of other top institutes.

William Shapiro, head of neuro-oncology at Memorial Sloan Kettering Cancer Institute in New York City, had agreed to become BNI's new chief of neurology. His acceptance meant prestige for that now-undistinguished department. Today he would clear up paper work and prepare for a meeting next week on the sea change about to take place here.

Everything was coming together, as he knew it must. The operation on Timmy Mathias had made headlines around the world, overshadowing the two standstills that showcased Barrow's strengths but in some ways just as reflective of those strengths, representing cooperation among disciplines. Rekate, the pediatric neurosurgeon, Sonntag, the spine expert, Spetzler, the master of the imaginative approach, had teamed up to do what would have been impossible for any one of them, just as the neurosurgeons of BNI had teamed with neuroanesthesiologists and St. Joseph's cardiovascular experts this morning for the second time this week.

Spetzler had spent half an hour on the phone yesterday with a reporter from the Soviet news agency, Tass, and been interviewed in German by reporters from Berlin to Vienna. While others had expressed fear over the outcome of the Mathias surgery, he had felt certain that once the boy survived the surgery without new injury, he would recover. The next morning, though still unresponsive to the residents commands, the boy had moved spontaneously on both sides, a good indicator that his brain stem was not irreparably damaged on either side.

Spetzler's skills in bringing patients through surgeries that few had ever survived were leading to an increasing number of invitations to present his cases at national and international meetings, and he was charismatic in those presentations; he loomed self-confident in a field of self-confident men. He had felt sure he was making the right move when John Green persuaded him to come here; now he knew it.

But how *had* Green pulled off that trick? The answer was the key to the next leap forward.

By the early 1980s, Green had built Barrow into an excellent institute—well endowed and nationally known. But not powerful, not influential. Green's own reputation as a neurosurgeon was secure; he would win a place in *Modern Neurosurgical Giants*, Paul Bucy's sequel to the volume on the founders of neurosurgery that dealt with the next generation. And Green had assembled a neurosurgical partnership of unquestioned excellence. BNI could rank with the best in patient care—that is, in morbidity and mortality.

But there was also no question that BNI had not reached the company of the handful of premier neurological institutes in the country, and now UCLA had a brain research institute as well as vast neurological capabilities, and was part of a major university, always touted as a requisite to world-class ranking in medicine. Green did not think the university connection was critical.

BNI's weak spots were in the remaining two criteria for measuring institutional excellence. The research program was good, but it lacked a fire-brand to give it direction. And in education, the third pillar of medicine, BNI carried out good residency training, but with no aspiration beyond training community neurosurgeons. To be viewed with the top institutes, you had to turn out academic neurosurgeons—future chairs and pioneers—as well as the physicians who would go into private practice in their communities. BNI was not looked to in any sense for peer education or for breakthroughs.

What got Spetzler to accept a job in territory Charles Wilson told him was "a wasteland, culturally and every other way"? What brought him to gamble his legacy on a place Wilson said "wouldn't be ashes without him"? Money. Not money for Spetzler's pocket. Money for research. John Green employed his silver-tongued oratory one more time to persuade the BNI fund-raising board that a well-endowed chair would give a top young neurosurgeon the one thing that he had to have, the freedom to build a program to match his own skills.

The board raised $1 million, the income from which provides in-house research funds to be used entirely at the director's discretion. The largest share of that $1 million came from an Oklahoma physician retired in the Valley, J. M. Harbor, and the chair was dedicated in his name. More funds were raised to build laboratory space. And from the neurosurgery partnership there was an income guarantee that is now more than $200,000. That meant that if the director spent a year without performing a single surgery, he would get that salary. On the other hand, Green rightly suspected that the guarantee would not matter, that the director would earn well over that figure on his own, and that was not a trifling matter.

The one drawback to academic medicine was that there usually were ceilings on the income that physician-professors could earn. That was true at Harvard, Columbia, virtually every major program in the country. Because the professors were part of an academic unit, their income beyond the ceiling was expected to support the institution. The surgery department was a major money-maker for any medical school, as was radiology; medicine and pediatrics, for example, were major money-losers. Academia was not supposed to be a place for a doctor to become wealthy.

These are not starvation wages, but consider that neurosurgeons' fees in most cases are in the thousands of dollars—around $5,000 recently—and most top brain surgeons operate on several cases a day, several days a week regardless of leadership and administrative duties or meetings. Million-dollar annual salaries are not unusual. According to the most recent figures compiled by the Center for Research in Ambulatory Health Care Administration, neurosurgeons' median income in 1989 was $341,950, meaning that half of all neurological surgeons earned more that year and half earned less. That amount was the highest of any medical specialty, just ahead of that of cardiovascular surgeons at $338,640. The earnings include those of academic neurosurgeons, most of whom earn far less than the median.

Spetzler left Case Western Reserve with no misgivings and even a sense of relief. "I interviewed all over the country," he said later. "I interviewed for a chairmanship in the D.C. area, and in New York. I came away from the East positively depressed with the state of affairs in neurosurgery." In part it was the overheated malpractice situation. "Some of the chairmen back there have more than a million dollars in suits in litigation. You can hardly feel professional satisfaction working under those circumstances."

But in part it was just the living and working climate of the East that Spetzler found disagreeable. An outdoorsman, ravenous skier, scuba diver, tennis player, swimmer, Spetzler found nothing to complain of in Phoenix.

Spetzler became chair of neurosurgery in 1983, director of Barrow on Green's retirement in 1986.

Academia was not the place to become wealthy, but it was the traditionally accepted place to create a legacy. There are two ways for a neurosurgeon to do so. First, as in all medicine, by building political power. That means winning leadership roles in the major national organizations, the American Association of Neurological Surgeons (the former Harvey Cushing Society), The Congress of Neurological Surgeons or the American Academy of Neurosurgeons. Second, by training the next generation of neurosurgical stars, that is, by running one of the country's top residency programs.

Spetzler chose the latter—although, to those who chose the former and are in positions of power, it was a choice luckily made, given his propensity for sharp comment. His friend Bennett Stein of Columbia says, "We're all a bunch of ego-maniacs. We all get up and say, 'Look what I can do.' But when you get up and say to us, 'Look what I can do that you can't do,' a lot of people take it badly. I don't. I welcome an argument. But if Robert does decide to take a national-leadership role, or to assume the chairmanship at one of the top institutions, he's going to have to tone down a little. The way he's got things going at Barrow, of course, I'm not sure why he'd want to."

Consider the Academy of Neurological Surgeons. To some, this is the highest circle of neurosurgical political power in America, to others the epitome of Good Old Boy elitism. Spetzler has been blackballed twice. Says one member, "He just pisses people off."

Meanwhile, Spetzler's reputation for consummate skill and intrepidity was growing rapidly. He was presenting an increasing number of complex cases at national meetings, and now internationally. While neurosurgeons around the country struggled to perfect the use of hypothermic arrest and deep barbiturate coma as a means to reach deep blood-vessel lesions, he was having a string of good outcomes. This coming summer he would go on sabbatical, first to London, on to Russia and finally to Vienna for two major projects that were indicators of his growing stature.

A few years earlier, he and Wolfgang Koos, head of neurosurgery at the University of Vienna and an old friend and mentor, had put out *A Color Atlas of Microneurosurgery*, which had rapidly become an international standard in the years following the introduction of the intraoperative microscope. He had known Koos since his student days in Munich and Switzerland, studying with *the* microneurosurgery pioneer, Gazi Yasargil. Now Spetzler and Koos would work on their second edition.

But what of Barrow's reputation? One of Spetzler's own top hands had put the problem this way, in assessing what Spetzler aimed to do for BNI's reputation: "It's one thing to amass a string of brilliant surgeries, to build a reputation as a leader in vascular neurosurgery, which absolutely without doubt he is. But it's quite another thing to bring that kind of reputation to an institute you head."

And consider the competition and the presumed peers.

New York City has six separate neurosurgical residency programs, all university-affiliated, three headed by national leaders in neurosurgery: Bennett Stein of Columbia University at the Neurological Institute, Leonard Malis at Mount Sinai School of Medicine at Mount Sinai Hospital, and Joseph Ransohoff at New York University at Bellevue.

Boston has three neurosurgical residencies and the Cushing legacy. Two are Harvard-based, at Brigham chaired by Peter Black, and at Massachusetts General Hospital headed by Nicholas Zervas. The program at New England Medical Center is headed by William Shucart of Tufts.

The University of California at San Francisco is the medical campus for the state's world-renowned public university system.

Research? Consider the names of the affiliate universities.

Neurosurgical stars? Zervas jokingly complained that he keeps losing his. "They keep running off to chair other nationally ranked programs." Robert Crowell to Illinois, though he later returned. Roberto Heros to Minnesota. Peter Black himself to Brigham. Get the picture?

National leadership? MGH's Robert Ojemann is the only person to have been president of all three major neurosurgical associations.

Not that everything is as it appears on paper. Spetzler always recognized that institutional reputations were evanescent, but appeared permanent. For years after a program had gone into decline, it would be touted as the best in the country, and because the top residents would continue choosing it for a time, the after-image would remain. On the other hand, for years after an institution had jammed shoulder to shoulder with the best, it would not have the luster of reputation; people would not think of it when asked to name the best. He was utterly convinced that that was Barrow's position, and that was frustrating. But it was solvable.

Spetzler drew highly ranked residents because of his own reputation. But to consistently bring in the best and brightest required an institutional commitment to research. This required a strong department of neurology, a service which here had no national leaders and no research agenda. Joseph White, an excellent physician, had no ambitions for national acclaim in neurology. He was ill and looking for ways to ease back, not gear up. By comparison, heading neuropathology was Peter Johnson, the only such specialist board certified in the state, who had a glowing academic record from Minnesota. John Hodak was as good as they come in neuroradiology, Burton Drayer was a national leader in neuroimaging.

Today he was putting the finishing touches on William Shapiro's arrival within months to take over neurology. Here was the major figure everyone had talked of. Shapiro was a renowned researcher and held an endowed chair at Memorial Sloan Kettering Cancer Institute in New York, certainly one of the country's top cancer centers. He was seasoned—in his early 50s—but still young enough to carry out major ambitions in neurological research. And he was ambitious in a very major way, admitting to no small frustration at not being able to carry out the broad programs of clinical investigations in all areas of brain research, not just cancer. Shapiro had bumped against the very confinement Spetzler had seen in major national institutions: too many hot-shots competing for resources. Shapiro wanted to get programs going in epilepsy, and there was Parkinsonism, there was Alzheimer's, there was—enthusiasm and drive. His wife, Joan, also was a noted brain researcher, a geneticist, who would run the cancer research laboratory.

To get Shapiro, Spetzler applied the same formula Green had used on him, promising state of the art laboratory space, including a lab for Joan Shapiro, an endowed professorship to guarantee research freedom, and room to maneuver. This professorship, as it turned out, bore a name far better known in Arizona than the J. M. Harbor of Spetzler's chair, and among journalists the most notorious name in the state: Kemper Marley.

Marley had always been identified in the media as a "liquor magnate," and newspaper accounts of his activities said he had been associated with bootleggers during prohibition and known-gangsters since. He was a tough old westerner and quick to shoot off his mouth at those he did not like, but the media have fawned over such characters under many circumstances. Not this time. *Arizona Republic* reporter Don Bolles was killed by a car bomb in 1976, and three men were tried and convicted for actually setting off the bomb; but who paid them? From the first, many sources, from police informants to investigative reporters, claimed in print that Marley was the still-unknown figure who paid for the killing, though Marley denied any connection to the murder or knowledge of it.

Did Spetzler have second thoughts about naming the Kemper and Ethyl Marley Chair in Neurology? "Not one," he said later. "First, I have absolutely nothing to say about his guilt or innocence, obviously. I did meet him, and found him quite likable, a rough-and-ready character. But the history of the United States is full of characters with less than savory pasts, appending their names to quite legitimate, even illustrious institutions—starting with John D. Rockefeller and the robber barons."

The $1 million endowment would allow Shapiro to move forward as Spetzler had, to turn neurology from an adequate residency for community neurologists into a top national residence for future academic neurologists. To do so without university ties required that large research commitment in-house. The endowment on the Harbor chair now had grown to $1.3 million, and Spetzler put every cent of the income into research—laboratory equipment, grants and the critical seed grants that allowed the researchers in James Bloedel's department of neurobiology to establish footholds in critical research areas that would enable them to get large and even multiyear federal grants.

"Only in the past five years has BNI emerged in the teaching field," Spetzler had told an interviewer. "And this means residency training, peer training. To find this outside the academic setting is extremely unusual. Now this is one of the top places that medical students apply to for residency."

Research. Neurosurgery was much about research. On the shelf above his secretary's desk stood file boxes containing his publications. The two right-most boxes read, "Dr. Spetzler's Publications 246-282" and "Dr. Spetzler's In Press 283-303." And not one sole authorship, that was the key. On every publication was a chain of names, of collaborators. Initially they were the names of his mentors, guiding him into the complexities of the vasculature. Then the other names came along, sometimes half a dozen or more, representing his junior colleagues, men and women now well-known in their own right, then his residents and fellows. The power of BNI would emanate from the residents, as they moved upward, and that movement would be empowered to a large extent by the amount and quality of the research they would do here.

That was one side of the training system, research and publication.

The phone rang. He glanced up at the monitor. It was time to return to the Jennifer Turner standstill.

Neurosurgery was most of all not *about* anything; it was *doing* neurosurgery, a broad name for some of the most complex and precisely coordinated perceptions, motions, and judgments humans had ever woven together. The standstill that drew so much attention hardly hinted at the complexity, and learning the complexity was what seven years' training was all about. That was the heart of the system as Cushing carried it into the new specialty of neurosurgery. And it was the system for which Spetzler felt and freely expressed much open contempt.

The creators of the system, Spetzler always says, were cruel, pitiless, hard, ego-driven. *They were not warm human beings.*

They punished their staffs, they were inhumane in their treatment of those they trained. They were supreme autocrats who could tolerate no flaw or mistake. And they unfortunately passed that on to many of those who came after.

Of The Founder, Spetzler has said, "Cushing was intolerant of the people who were residents. He took the attitude of treating them as lesser human beings. He addressed them as underlings, and then once in a while to make up for it given them the pat on back, or invited them for tennis or dinner.

"But it was an abusive system, and that carried over for many years. There are currently still a significant number of individuals who are in training positions carrying out that philosophy." Indeed, in terms of being hard drivers and accepting no flaw, no error, more of the top chairs appear to be of the Cushing School than the Spetzler. But he says, "It's a philosophy I personally couldn't be more diametrically opposed to, a philosophy I've found exceedingly distasteful whenever I've encountered it."

He headed out past the residents' library, out the offices' back door to the elevator inside St. Joseph's main entrance on Thomas Road, back to OR 1.

THE CUSHING SCHOOL. Here is Charles Wilson: of medium height, wiry as advertised, jet black hair, part Cherokee Indian on his mother's side and shows it in his chiseled, angular features and dark complexion. Son of a small-town druggist but his father was not his major influence. "My mother set my motor running on high," he says. "The more time goes by, the more apparent that is." He readily admits that having to be the best at everything is a driving compulsion with him. "If I was a butterfly collector," he says with a twang of Oklahoma still in his voice, "I'd have to have the best butterfly collection in the world. First in the United States. But eventually in the world."

Totally dedicated. No life outside neurosurgery—recently divorced from his fourth wife. Wears running shoes at all times in the hospital for good reason: He sometimes has four ORs going at once.

He has run half a dozen marathons, including Boston and New York. A tough, hard man. "I don't know how else to be," he says. "I just can't coddle people. I don't know how to put things easy when life and death are at stake."

He has a harsh reputation for firing residents in a profession where that is rare, for being intolerant of any flaw and any error, yet in the operating room supremely patient, never loses it, never rages.

Given that his standards are so high for accepting residents, doesn't he feel he loses good people when a high percentage are forced to leave—some say as high as 25 percent. "Obviously not, or I wouldn't do it."

And he can take it as good as he gives it out. At a birthday party roast

Robert himself proposed that Wilson's residents had worries over their job security, but they were better off than his wives. You see why the top chairs of neurosurgery call *each other* arrogant and aggressive, and what they mean by that. They are utter perfectionists and believers in the axiom, Show me a good loser and I'll show you a loser.

Ask Bennett Stein, who is certainly one of the great chairmen, to name the great chairmen—because that is to name the top programs in neurosurgery in this period when Spetzler is still reaching.

He rattles off Wilson, Joe Ransohoff of NYU, John Jane of Virginia, Donlin Long of Johns Hopkins, all men of his own generation, now in or near the decade of their retirement.

Look at Ransohoff. He is seventy-three years old and looks nearer sixty, lean and mean and wiry as the college lightweight boxer he was until somebody rearranged his face, still sporting the bicep tattoo he got back then. His wife is younger than several of his grandchildren, as he points out, and the couple's picture is prominent on his office wall, she very pregnant in a bikini, he grinning broadly, his hand on her belly. The boy is a toddler now. Ransohoff wears cowboy boots and jeans under his green-scrub top and chain smokes cigarettes—though in the three years between two interviews he switched to a low-tar brand. Does 100 pushups and swims every day.

Is it fair to say Ransohoff is of the Cushing School?

"Are you kidding!" He thrusts out his forearms. "Looka me!"

He turned a fallen down program in decrepit Bellevue Hospital into a nationally first-rate residency. That's what wild men do. Hung on there so long—too long, Stein says—that Eugene Flam gave up waiting to take over and went to Penn. (And there's another wild man.)

Stein says when the great Lawrence Poole retired from Columbia thirty years ago, Ransohoff was the logical choice to replace him. "But they were afraid of Joe, too strong willed, too determined, so they hired a non-entity, who was my predecessor." *Sayonara*, whoever that was. Stein on his own doesn't mention MGH, whose program is run by Zervas, politically one of the most powerful men in neurosurgery and whose department includes Robert Ojemann, not only one of the country's premier neurosurgeons by acclamation, but perhaps politically the most powerful in the country.

What about MGH's program?

"Mediocre," Stein says. "Too uppity. Too Harvard." Now Charles Wilson at UCSF, there is Stein's and everybody's idea of somebody who created something out of nothing. "It was *nothing* when he got there. Now it's one of the top in the country. Maybe *the* top."

Everybody has something to say about Charlie Wilson. Peter Black, one of the most thoughtful, least caustic of these chairmen, says, "I think Charlie Wilson is one of the most complex and fascinating men in the world. And I'm not sure you'll ever get to the bottom of him. But what a program he's created!" And Black does think MGH is one of the nation's tops. "Nick Zervas has done something marvelous. He's surrounded himself with people who are great. Bob Ojemann, Bob Crowell. And the chairmen who've come out of his program!" Black, self-effacing, does not mention himself as he lists the MGH legacy.

And that's the kind of greatness Black lays to Charlie Wilson: not only the drive, the boundless energy, but the ego-strength to surround himself with people good enough to beat him. For in final judgment of the top people, who you mold is the final measure of just how good you were.

Physically prepossessing men—and all men, so far. Thor Sundt, who heads neurosurgery at the Mayo Clinic, was a West Point graduate and decorated infantryman in Korea. He was featured on CBS's "Sixty Minutes" because, in the throes of colon cancer, he continues to operate regularly. Roberto Heros, of the younger generation, got his baptism of fire on the beach at the Bay of Pigs.

Spetzler says of the Wilson legacy, "When I took over the BNI, I decided I would devote myself to the residency program; that would be the way I would build the excellence of the institution. As a chairman I would be expected to take part in national organizations as a leader—as a president, a conference organizer. Instead I participate as a presenter. I have put all that energy into the residency program. That was something I learned from Charlie Wilson."

Because that's what he did?

"Because that's what he didn't do. And I decided I would."

And that's where Spetzler is coming from. Not only in the OR, but on rounds every afternoon at 4:30 or 5:30 or whenever his surgeries and the other business of the day are done, any day he is not on the road.

Spetzler rounds. In the darkened Radiology Suite, crowded in the small room adjoining the the giant torus of the CT scanner, the residents and fellows crowd close in the darkness with the only illumination coming from the wall panels where, in angiograms, arteries coming wriggling out aglow, twisting, branching, concealing all but the faintest hint of aneurysm or bleeding or malformation. Or they look at MRI and CT scans, where the hemispheres of the cerebrum swell up out of the brain stem, over the cerebellum, as startlingly realistic as at autopsy and looking at first glance like all cerebrums, unindividuated. But now, here, look down into the left lateral ventricle, that cave just above the rind of the corpus callosum joining the two hemispheres, that cave whose walls drip out cerebrospinal fluid and where the fluid collects to be drained as it is replenished.

Anything unusual there?

No. Midline looks okay between left and right lateral ventricles.

Santa Grazia! Holy Mother Moses. You call that all right?

Another voice: *There looks to be slight displacement of the left ventricle, in the anterior horn.*

Due to? Due to?

He calls on them by name, residents, fellows, interns, tries to remember names even of the visiting medical students, although he has a terrible memory for names. It's the only obvious fault in his intelligence and it drives him nuts.

By contrast, by consensus, you would be proud of yourself if Charlie Wilson remembered your name by your third year of residency. The tough guys have a lot of history going for them. But Spetzler sees another way. The control of Wilson, leavened with visible warmth and humor. The fellows here, who have done their residency training with others, all describe a shock getting used to Spetzler's friendliness. Does he remember the residents' names? They play tennis at his house! They drop in, swim and relax there!

One time a bunch of residents were there helping Spetzler put up or take down his storm windows, the Boss himself doing the homeowner routine.

Suddenly the window slipped in his grip and his right hand went right through the pane. There was blood everywhere and a huge dagger of glass stuck right through Spetzler's right forearm. His right forearm. Everybody looked near panic. Spetzler grabbed the glass dagger, pulled it out, then held up his arm and flexed his fingers. Instantly he broke into that big grin. "No problem," he said.

Who knows if Charlie Wilson takes down storm windows? He runs, runs, runs with no break. Who sees Joe Ransohoff being a klutz with storm windows? Spetzler is personable. He really likes people. And that has a role here, and is part of an aim that is clear.

But will it work? That is, one can envision fine neurosurgeons pouring forth from Spetzler's program, humane and skilled, taking their places in operating rooms around the country. But will they take their places in professorships at leading neurological institutes? Will they eventually move into key chairmanships where they will beget the next generation of neurosurgeons who trace lineage to Robert Spetzler? He is aiming for nothing less than that. And he is aware, as all people are whose reputation derives from physical powers, of his own mortality, of how little time a chairman has to make his mark in "a career that is really half a career," as he often says. If such believing in one's destiny is arrogance, then he is arrogant; for he does believe.

THE ART OF DOING MANY THINGS at once was the first thing new residents had to learn. After they learned to do many things at once, they had to learn to stop and concentrate absolutely on only one thing, for a measurable time but for a time that might seem forever.

Pressure transforms craft into art, and when the pressure is on time it can compress a string of events, be they musical or otherwise, until they overlap one another—in resonance and harmony for the skillful, at odds and in cacophony for those who fail.

The simplest such overlaps in music are rounds, those familiar songs whose singers begin the same simple tune, repeating it over and over, usually after a time delay, as in, "Row, row, row your boat," and now the second voice, "Row, row, row your...." And so on. There was much of that from day to day in the lie of a resident. Most of what the residents did was not complicated, looked at in isolation. But it was not in isolation; on and on it went, growing ever more complicated as parts of each string of chores had to be done at the same time as different parts of the same chore for a different patient. Not precisely the same time, of course, but close enough.

A canon is based on the same idea as a round, but is much more complex, because the second voice coming in is singing a variation on the theme, not a true copy but perhaps an octave higher, or with the melody reversed. The tough part for the composer is that the *single sound* produced at any given moment by, say, three notes coming from three different parts, has to sound good. *Has to sound good.* Follow the rules and sound good. And that's how it went here, at a higher level. Residents must follow the rules, without deviation, learn and follow the rules, though which rule might apply at which moment grew more difficult. What corresponds to sounding good? In following the rules, everything had to end up hanging together. It did no good to show you could follow the rules if everything fell apart and patients died or sickened, or no one got admitted on time for surgery, or you didn't make it to the ER in time to examine a trauma patient for head or neck injury.

And finally there is the fugue, the most complex of the three that follow this same idea of introducing higher-level repeats that are not quite repeats. The fugue, too, goes on and on, with a newly entering musical voice overlaying a theme so similar to the preceding that it catches your ear, your mind's ear. And endless in repetition it is, and not quite a repetition, now faster, now slower, and sometimes working in upon itself.

But unlike the canon, which is very rigid, the fugue has no rules. That's why it's the most complex. Anything goes, or, anything can go *if it can be made to go.* And hangs together. And maybe that's how neurosurgery is, in the end. After learning all the increasingly-more complex rules and learning to play them in every variation, you come to places where not all of the rules apply, and you are not absolutely bound to follow those that do. Because now the only rule is that everything *absolutely* has to hang together. Now the only standard is outcome. Residents do not perform fugues; they do rounds, play their parts in the canons, and aspire to the fugues.

seven

Rounds

SATURDAY–SUNDAY
MAY

BARROW NEUROLOGICAL INSTITUTE
NEUROSURGERY ASSIGNMENTS AND SERVICE

WEEKEND AND HOLIDAY ICU ROUNDS

Rounds will begin at 0730 in Radiology. Notes are
to be written on all ICU patients by all residents on call
(both departing and oncoming residents).

Floor patients will be seen by the oncoming and
departing first tier residents.... The senior resident
on call will be contacted by the resident after the patients
have been seen if any problems arise.

WEEKENDS WERE TRAUMA TIME. Head-injuries come
in from boat crashes on the Colorado, from sand-rail collisions beyond in
California's Algodones Dunes, rollovers on the Navajo Reservation at the four
corners Arizona forms with Utah, Colorado and New Mexico, from urban
head-ons and strokes in the desert, and of course from shootings, knifings,
beatings and God knows what else. St. Joe's did not get the same volume
of trauma as the county hospital, but it and the UA were the only Level 1—

most serious—neuro trauma units in all Arizona and for a good bit of the bordering counties of neighbor states. Weekend call was different from weekday call; there was more trauma but less of everything else that dogged a junior resident's life.

Jennifer Turner slipped in and out of normal consciousness. Within two days of surgery, when she should still have been deep in the effects of barbiturate coma, she was clamoring to get out of bed. Yet she still had intermittent double vision. Perhaps that was only an indication that the optic nerve had been jarred as the neurosurgeons worked toward the front of her brain stem, but perhaps it was a more serious sign that brain swelling was pressing down onto one or both optic nerves.

Millions of light-receptor nerve endings dot the back of the retina in a continuous matrix and bundle there into the large optic nerve, then stream out the optic canal through one of the five fused bones of the eye orbit. The left and right nerve bundles run along the base of the brain hemispheres until they reach the circle of Willis. Dead center in that circle, the pituitary gland hangs down like a soft nodule. The twin optic nerves then perform a dazzling interchange. Within the circle, they cross over in an X just ahead of the pituitary, then head rearward toward a variety of brain structures, mostly in the occipital lobes at the rear. Because the optic nerve and the three other cranial nerves involved in eye motion travel through such "high-value real estate," any unusual eye responses after brain surgery bear close watching as messengers of what is happening within.

JENNIFER WOULD BECOME AGITATED and impatient to leave, then lethargic. Double vision came and went. She still had not seen her son. "I don't want him to see me here like this," she told her mother. "I've got to get home."

Then, on the night of Mother's Day, she had a strange dream. She was having a party, thrown for her by the hospital attendants, everyone feeling fine and being very friendly to her. Unusually friendly. She headed down the hall to find a bathroom and suddenly realized there was no party, it was just a dream. But now she was wide awake and really was heading down a darkened hallway, in a ward that was eerily deserted. Most of the beds were unmade. She had no idea how she had gotten here but suddenly her head began to throb, there again. She was headed for this ward, she knew. And as she realized that, and realized why, the old chill returned. She was freezing.

The beds were unmade, the mattresses' ticking was striped and dull as death. They were going to bring her here to kill her. Why? She was terrified even more than she had been before the surgery. *They're going to kill me. Then I'll be put in a bag on one of these unmade beds.* She wandered toward a double door at the end of the ward, but she couldn't get to it. "Help! Please, someone help me," she said in as calm a voice as she could manage. And then she woke up. She felt fine; her mother and grandmother were there at her bedside. The sun was out. No headache, no chills. It was early on a gorgeous morning in May.

And then came the swirl of white coats, greetings all around, as eight residents on their rounds filled the small room. The one in charge, a black man of medium height, began reading from her chart. Once he passed "Jennifer Turner, seventeen days post-op," she couldn't follow a word he said, but by the way they all smiled and nodded it sounded good. Finally, he said, "Looks like you'll be going home soon."

FRED WILLIAMS LED THE THRONG through the ICU alone, since Tom Grahm had to scrub in for surgery. He would do this for only two months longer, when his residency would end. The son and younger brother of doctors, he had had no illusions about the grind he faced when he had decided to become a neurosurgeon, though in many ways it was not as bad as advertised. When his father checked in as a resident, he basically lived in the hospital for the duration and was not paid enough to live anywhere else, anyway.

Williams and Grahm each earned $35,000 a year, compared to the junior residents' $30,000. The fellows earned only about $40,000. None of it was what anyone thought of as physicians' wages, let alone brain surgeons'. Still, it was enough income for Williams and his wife and two daughters to live in a comfortable apartment. In a few months he would become one of only about two dozen black neurosurgeons in the country, but it was a small specialty. He had been hired as an assistant professor at the Arizona College of Medicine, his first job an academic appointment. Of more than

600,000 licensed physicians in the United States, only 4,300 are neuro-surgeons. By comparison, three times that number specialize in cardio-vascular surgery, also not a large specialty. Nearly 100,000 physicians are in internal medicine and nearly 40,000 in general surgery.

Williams's stars had not always seemed so lucky. With his older brother training to be an ophthalmologist, like their father, Fred had done early training as a hellion. Took several years to get an AA degree in mathematics in San Francisco. Borrowed his brother's new sports car and, with the admonition to be careful ringing in his ears, took it full tilt down a winding canyon road. Made all but one of the hairpins, sailing off a curve, turning 180 degrees, landing thirty or so feet below in the canyon. Car totaled. Fred unhurt. But a bit chastened as a wild man. On now to the University of California, Irvine, where he graduated *summa cum laude,* and he had continued to earn honors in medical school.

Onward. The morning sun cleared the neighboring rooftops and distant Squaw Peak, to glint in their eyes as they moved from room to room down the polished corridor of the ICU. All the hallway walls are glass from waist-level up, so patients in distress are visible to anyone traveling through. In addition, monitors at the nursing station show all patients not directly visible from there.

"Patient ..."

Jack Schulte, sixty-four-year-old male, nineteen days post-op following hypothermic arrest with induced barbiturate coma for basilar tip aneurysm. He sleeps peacefully, coming around far more slowly than Jennifer Turner, but his age was not in his favor. Wife Shirley smiled up as the residents closed in around his bed. Jack has a pleasant, round face and a fringe of graying hair. On the walls are get-wells from children and grandchildren, pictures of all of them and several pictures of his favorite granddaughter, whom he calls "Weenie" to tease her—since she, like her friends, uses that word to describe other kids who annoy her. So now it's become kind of a secret word between them as she turns fourteen.

Blood pressure a little high, blood gases—basically meaning the oxygen and carbon dioxide balance of respiration—are good. It will take longer to know if he will recover completely or not. But Shirley believes he is rising steadily, if slowly. "Some days I'm sure he's following every word I say, but he's just deciding to stay within himself," she says. "Sometimes I think he's tuning me out. He's saying, 'I don't think I'm going to be bothered today.'"

Shirley had been a popular singer in little theater over the years back in Cincinnati. And even little theater required an enormous devotion of time and energy, especially while raising a family. While she acted and sang, Jack did carpentry for the troupe—always loved carpentry.

At this word, his eyes look over at her and he smiles faintly. "See what I mean?" she says, cheered. "All those years, I was the one who was out front, getting to do what I wanted. Jack never complained about being in the background, about not getting the attention. Now I figure it's his turn."

Jack and Shirley had retired a few years ago to Sun City, west of Phoenix. They loved it. Everyone was family there. Jack built gorgeous cherry wood Early American reproductions in the community center wood shop. Shirley sang in the church choir and did many solo parts; her soprano voice had held strong and true. Each Easter she sang the solo in "Hallelujah," by Gaither and Huff, Jack's favorite.

Again he smiled. Was it a smile of recognition? The return of a full memory, of awakening self? Or was it a reflexive smile at a word that sat like the tip of an iceberg above a whole world of relations that would not come back?

Just the other day, Jack got another card signed by "Weenie." "And when I told him that, he really smiled." And indeed, he really smiles again, like someone distracted, staring a bit vacantly as though interrupted while musing on something that has little to do with the sensoria pouring in through our eyes here, suddenly smiling when brought back, then off again.

People make incredible comebacks from neurological injury. Comatose for years, they suddenly blink and come around. Or even more often, move as Jack Schulte seems to be moving, from blur to resolution. The patient moving from superficially responsive, like this, to more alert, to articulate. Articulation. Discrimination. Resolution. That can take hours, as for Jennifer, weeks, months, even years. But plainly he is not comatose in the traditional sense. He is GCS 8; he is beginning to respond to commands, sometimes.

The white-coated troop plunges groundward now, spirals down the stairwell to the second-floor trauma ICU. There new litanies are recounted, of accident, terror, termination of normal life; mixed in with the optimistic prognoses, leavened with the glory of a near-miss: "You're in good shape Mr. J. You're going out to the floor today, and you'll be home within a week! Who'd have believed that two weeks ago, 'ey?"

On down to the last stop, and the one they had dread the most just a few weeks ago, Pediatrics ICU. "You've heard about the Mathias kid?" And of course everyone had. He is not in a room but out on the floor of the ICU, where he can be watched more closely, where no one can sit, pass by, open the refrigerator holding medications without seeing him and his electronic monitors. But it seems an inappropriate place, in the middle of all this traffic, to see the high bed, the body almost entirely encased in white, with one leg raised. The cruel black-steel halo brace with its black crown pressed into the boy's skull; his eyes were blackened and his face scraped.

Kerry Mathias sits by the bed; she naps here, sleeps in the waiting room, very occasionally goes home but not for long. She is toughing it out.

"Let's see," Williams says gently. "How's Timmy doing this morning."

Brian Fitzpatrick reads that he is now over two weeks postop. Fitzpatrick is assigned to the pediatric service for these six months, so he is TJ's primary doctor, with Rekate the attending physician. Vital signs are good. Still does not show much of a Glasgow Coma Scale reading. Papadapolous' research has confirmed what they thought at the outset: no cases to match this in the literature. Complete clean fracture of the C1 vertebra holding neck to skull base. Those cases only reached the emergency room in two ways. Most frequently, dead. Very occasionally, someone would be brought in, somewhere in the world, who had not suffered any injury beyond the fracture—no hemorrhaging—and who had been immobilized at the scene, as Timmy was. A couple of those people recovered.

He was now off respirator and breathing on his own, an excellent sign. Blood gases normal.

Then Fitzpatrick systematically began the Glasgow Coma test. "Timmy, this is Dr. Fitzpatrick. Can you hear me Timmy?" Nothing.

Kerry tries: "TJ, Mommy's here. Can you hear me, sweetheart? Mommy's here." Nothing.

But as Fitzpatrick lightly pinched the boy's chest on the left, TJ's hand suddenly wavered upward toward the pain. He tried the other side. A little paralysis there, but some motions. Murmuring among the crowd. "This is a good sign, Mrs. Mathias," Williams said, carefully, carefully. "That he should be reacting like this so soon is very good."

But out in the hallway, down still another flight, there was an excited tone in their voices they couldn't allow themselves in front of the mother. Anything could still go wrong, ruin all the hopeful signs; dragging everyone down again. But he was localizing to pain.

Consider: The motor cortex, the neurons of voluntary movement, sits high up in the cerebrum just at the juncture of the parietal lobe at the crown and the frontal lobe. The left hemisphere controls the right side of the body; the right controls the left. Before controlling anything, all the cabling from those neurons passes down through the midbrain, down through the brain stem, each level downward representing increasingly automatic movements, down to the conditioned reflexes, to head down through the foramen magnum, the hole in the base of the brain, to become the fibers of the spinal cord. Damage the right side of the brain at any level, and the left side does not move; damage the left and you get paralysis on the right. Ten hours post-op, he had moved on both sides. But now he was not operating on primitive reflexes of withdrawal from pain or extending to it; he was reaching for the source of it.

PAUL FRANCIS PEELED OFF from the group and headed back up to the third floor to Sav-A-Day, the program that allowed patients to enter the hospital on the same day as their surgery instead of the night before, to save a day in billing. Today Francis was on first call and he hustled, knowing that dawn rounds marked the slowest his day would get. Francis was thirty-three years old, nearly six and a half feet tall with a somewhat sharp but long face, jet black hair, balding and, like all the residents but especially those on call, a determined look about him. He had had a vacation two months earlier, but what was wearing on him now was that he had not had a real weekend off in nearly two months.

He was on first call every third night, alternating with Bruce Cherny and whatever rotator was on the neurosurgical service at the time, the rotator being a resident in another specialty doing the obligatory period learning another area. That meant he came in this morning at the normal hour of five-thirty, put on scrubs and the personalized white coat of the neurosurgical service, and began his own bedside rounds. He was on Spetzler's service this month, meaning that all of the Boss's voluminous surgical caseload fell to him to check up on. Fitzpatrick, two years senior to him, had the Mathias boy as his responsibility, but he had a far smaller caseload in Peds (pronounced pedes) neurosurgery.

Today Paul Francis is also on first call. That means he must admit patients for neurosurgery today and tomorrow—endless paper work—handle emergencies and check treatments throughout the neurosurgery service, and most important, serve as the neurosurgery representative on the trauma team. As cases came in through the Emergency Room, it would be his job to check them for potential head or neck injury, and immediately call the next senior neurosurgeon in the tier if he had doubts or questions.

Here we are on 6 East for neurosurgical cases. Elise M., age sixty-seven, postop day six following surgery for arteriovascular malformation. "Good afternoon, Mrs. M———," Francis says. "How are you feeling today?" "Just fine. I'll be ready to go home soon I think," she says cheerfully."

"I'm sure you will. Can you tell me where you are now?" Broadly, a shared joke, "This is our daily game we play here on neuro rounds, and Mrs. M——— is one of my favorite players." She says she's in St. Joe's, in Phoenix. "And what day is today? Day and date? Right." He casts his eyes heavenward, a silly game but whatta ya gonna do. "And can you say this for me? Nelson Rockefeller drives—"

She completes the sentence, "—a Lincoln Continental," laughing. She recognizes nonsense.

" Mrs. M———, I want you to do rounds for me."

On down the hall. He questions each person routinely, no matter how alert they seem. Who is president of the United States? What city are you in? Amused or bored, they all answer.

Here is Emilio L———, a Hispanic man just twenty-one though he looks a few years older, with a friendly, engaging manner and a ready smile. Answers Francis's questions about his headaches, his doctor's diagnosis—

possible AVM. Raises his arms on command, follows Francis's moving finger with his eyes. Obviously a perfect 15. Francis leaves the room to get a blood pressure cuff and in the momentary awkwardness, Emilio nods toward the downtown area. "I just got in from the south."

Down by the border?

"Right," he nods vigorously and shakes his head. He looks around the window, checking the slanting shadows of sunlight to get his bearings. "Yeah, from the south. I came in by medevac."

A lot of people come in by helicopter.

"Right. They were shooting our guys down there."

Jesus! Drug shootout? What do you mean?

"No. They were shooting our guys. I was one of those going to be shot next but they got me out in time."

Perfect timing. Francis swoops in and begins. "Can you tell me what day today is, Mr. L——?"

"May 17."

"Right. And what city are you in?"

"What city?" He looks askance. "What do you mean what city. This is a field hospital isn't it?"

"I mean, where are you, Mr. L——? Where are we now?"

"In South Vietnam," he says, a curious smile playing on his face, trying to figure out if Francis is tricking him. "In the Republic of South Vietnam."

"Now? You're in Vietnam now?"

"Sure. The VC were shooting some of our guys. They just got me out in time."

In the hall, Francis says, "He was too young to have been in Vietnam; he was too young to have seen anything about Vietnam on television. Maybe an older brother, maybe his father." He shakes his head; there is an eeriness cast on the afternoon that won't be shaken loose. He seemed perfectly okay, GCS 15. An alert, responsive young man, genuinely glad to be alive after a near miss with death, on a battlefield that fell silent when he was a toddler. But the spell will not break easily, for here is the very next stop, up two flights and over from east corridor to west:

"Alan B——, male aged twenty-seven," he reads from the chart, "closed

head injury, possible closed skull fracture in fall from a moving car."
Closed injury meaning there is no opening in the scalp, therefore no immediate threat of infection. The man sits propped on his bed, his wife seated
next to him. He wears slacks but has a hospital gown on over them.
"What happened here, Mr. B ——?"

"Things that should've happened long ago," he says with a confident grin,
but his wife looks a bit rueful, though she smiles up at him supportively as he
continues. "I've been drinking too much, and generally not doing as I should.
But the Lord provides answers, and he's provided the answer now."

Alan's adored older brother has always hated him, he explains. Even said so.
Hated him because he, the brother, was sent to Vietnam and got all screwed
up, got ruined over there and came back on drugs and couldn't get his life
together. "And he said outright he hated me, because I didn't have to go and get
fucked up like he did. And I said, it's not my fault. What can I do about it?
Sometimes he was great, he was really great. He's my brother and I love him.
But then sometimes the meanness would come over him."

All the while he talks Francis writes, not Alan's words but the information
he will need for his H and P—history and physical—but the young man,
encouraged by what appears to be a taking of dictation, plows on.

"But anyway, I finally knew we had to have a showdown, that we had to
get together so I could tell him how I felt, how it wasn't my fault and I loved
him. He was going to be in town, and I was going to meet him and everything
was going to get straightened out. And I was drinking beers, probably too
many beers."

His wife is holding his hand now as he becomes more animated.

"How many beers?" Francis asks.

"About thirty."

"Thirty? *Thirty cans of beer?* In what period of time?"

"Since this morning. Since about ten this morning."

"So in about four hours you had thirty cans of beer?"

"Yes. But I wasn't driving. My wife drove and we went to meet my brother."

"And were you drinking then?'

"Yes, I had a beer with me in the car. And, anyway, when I saw my brother,
all of a sudden it came to me that things were going to work out. I saw him

there, and I knew I could talk to him and tell him and he wouldn't hate me anymore. And I got out of the car to go and meet him."

"And the car was still moving." Finally the picture is coming clearer.

"Yes." Alan laughs.

"At what speed was the car moving?"

Wife: "Forty miles an hour."

Francis has stopped writing. "So the car was moving at forty miles an hour, and you opened the door and stepped out?"

"Right! But that's the beautiful part of it. Maybe it took something like this. The Lord has strange ways to give us answers, but he gives us answers!" Sober as a judge, he sounds and looks. "And guess what? My brother said just what I said. He said he doesn't hate me anymore, and he's sorry. We need to start over again."

Down the corridor Francis plunges, as the brain weaves. How it weaves, labyrinths more wondrous than Daedelus's, called reality. And weaver of its own beholder, called mind. Or is it the other way around? Who is the weaver here, and who is the tapestry? The trauma bells rang again at 4 p.m. and the helicopter dropped in its tornado of dust, and later ambulances arrived from several accidents, and Francis napped in the residents' call room off 4ICU, periodically grabbing the ringing phone to answer questions from the floor or ICU about medications, vital signs. And then it was time for rounds again.

Through 4ICU, down to 2 ICU, over to Peds ICU.

THIS MORNING, as Kerry murmurs to TJ, his eyes open. He looks around; not at her, just looks around. The doctors initially think he might have cortical blindness—the eyes receiving and processing light normally, so that reflexes to light are normal, but the brain unable to process it. Frequently the cortically blind person holds images in the "mind's eye" that he or she believes are of the real world. The cortically blind person may falsely believe he can see. Even so, eye movements like this exhilarate his brain specialists. Involuntary eye movement is controlled by the cerebellum, working through the brain stem. Both eyes were moving together, looking all around, and for a time now TJ had been moving right and left arms and legs. The delicate and vital brain stem, somehow, had come all the way back, and so had its connections to the cerebellum, even though it was not completely certain that the links of vision remained in the occipital lobes.

Kerry and Tim had spent the first days after his surgery at the hospital, sleeping in a room reserved for families of very-critical children. Both gave up their jobs, one of them sitting with him constantly.

She is sure he hears and understands. Brian Fitzpatrick seems optimistic, but he is not so sure there's any recognition on TJ's part. Something remarkable is going on, he is sure of that.

On May 16, Spetzler addressed an auditorium full of journalists from around the world, all of whom had descended for whatever tidbit they could get, for whatever photo op might present itself, on TJ Mathias, the Miracle Child. The journalists ran the gamut from the principal U.S. wire services, leading dailies and local network outlets, to the respected German news weekly *Stern*, down to the supermarket tabloids (Boy Loses Head! Docs Put It Back On!).

Everyone from Fitzpatrick to Rekate and Sonntag was on pins and needles. The intensity of interest was frighteningly premature. The Miracle Child was still comatose, out, maybe GCS 8 at his best. And now, just when Rekate and Sonntag were their most worried that the popular press would misunderstand the uncertain nature of neurological recovery, up stepped the director.

"Timmy Mathias will not only recover all his neurological function completely," Spetzler said confidently. "He will walk out of St. Joseph's Hospital. I don't know when, but he will walk out of here."

Then, as Kerry came in at seven-thirty one morning toward the end of May, a nurse ran up to her with exciting news: "He spoke to us."

"What did he say?"

"He said, 'Please help me.'"

Monday
June

CALL SCHEDULE: First call will be covered by Drs. Francis, Cherny and second-tier residents. The call will be every third night for Drs. Francis and Cherny.

DICTATIONS: All ER consults, inpatient neurosurgery consults, admissions, procedures and discharge summaries must be dictated.

WEEKDAY ICU MORNING ROUNDS: All ICU patients will be seen
and notes written by the assigned resident prior to start of rounds
at 0630 Monday-Thursday and 0545 Friday. Residents should arrive
45 minutes prior to rounds to see patients.

MONDAY CONFERENCES: Pediatric Neurology/Neurosurgery
conference 0730.

BOB CUNNINGHAM, ONE OF TJ'S NURSES, left a teddy bear for him at
the foot of his bed, while everyone was still unsure if he was really "in" or not.

"I watched him reach for it with his toes, and pull it up to where he could
grab it with his hand," Cunningham told Fitzpatrick. "And then I knew he was
there all right."

Now this scene just a week or so later: TJ, propped in a wheelchair near the
nursing station, waiting for someone to take him to physical therapy. It's hard
to tell if he is aware of anything. At his foot is the teddy bear. A passing nurse
picks it up and puts it in his lap, continuing on. He suddenly grabs the
teddy bear and flings it, a good ten feet. He is an angry and bored ten-year-old.
He is in.

He had risen like a rocket from that first stare around him. Incomprehen-
sible whispers to his parents while he was still intubated had become hand
signals to let them know when he was in pain.

He is tall for his age, like his father's brothers. You can see his mother's
smile in his mischievous, elfin grin, and he has her eyes—they crinkle at the
corners when he smiles.

Betty Bolden, one of his therapists, had been surprised that he mastered
the balance board on his first try. Still in his leg cast, he'd had to balance
the board on a half cylinder, to keep it from rolling underneath him. "He is
a miracle child," Betty said, echoing the phrase used in news stories around
the world. But she means it literally.

"When I first saw him, before he was out of his coma, I thought God had
special plans for him," she said quietly. "Sometimes we need to see that miracles
still do happen." She and her husband put TJ on their "TLC" list for the church
prayer group they lead. In the mail, he has gotten an announcement of
perpetual prayer in his name, and, anonymously, a bottle of holy water.

He dotes on his sister, Rachel. "He's very protective of her," Kerry says.

Just before he went home, he lay dressed on his bed, awkwardly half-upright because of the halo brace, cradling Rachel in his arms. As she squirmed and wriggled, he chided, "Careful, Rachel, don't fall. You're gonna hurt yourself."

Where did he hear that warning? (Or Rachel hers, wagging her finger, in her perfect three-year-old's voice as TJ roars down the hall in his wheelchair: "No wheelies, TJ. No wheelies!")

Jack Schulte is not all the way back yet, but he continues to rise, and Shirley tells the rounding residents she is sure he is taking in more than he lets on, even now when he lets on more. He follows commands, when he feels like it, a sign that he is responsive to the environment. But to the residents "when he feels like it" does not add up to 15. He smiles when Shirley brings up people and things he likes. He nods in response. Plainly the fog is clearing.

The Schulte children arrived from Cincinnati and that seemed to make him brighter. Son Jerry, a field biologist with the firm contracted to clean up the Ohio River; daughter Gayla Parker, a fourth grade teacher. There with their spouses and children. One night Jack laughed at a comment Gayla made.

Schulte's surgery and hospital care at Barrow cost $108,249.88, covered by insurance; that was the bill as of May 27, when he was moved to the sixth floor, to begin rehabilitation. He was discharged at the end of June, more than two months after his surgery.

On discharge Jack and Shirley went to see George Prigatano, head of BNI's neuropsychiatry. He gave Jack a few tests designed to measure his awareness and concentration. When Prigatano drew two sides of a triangle, Schulte drew the third side. But when asked to draw a triangle, he could not. Analogous results were shown in further tests.

He could not initiate action, Prigatano said. It was called frontal lobe syndrome, and no one entirely understood it, but basically it meant he could follow commands and respond to questions, but he could not initiate activity on his own. The cause was damage to the frontal lobes, and although the controls of life resided far from there, much of what we consider personality and will derives from activity in this farthest reach of evolution's neural growth.

Unable to initiate. That was as opposite Jack as Shirley could imagine. But it was something. In the mornings when they awoke, she would ask him how he was and he would say, "Fine," in the same strong voice she remembered. If she joked, he laughed. They would build from there.

Back at St. Joseph's on this scorching summer morning, Bruce Cherny had not yet finished writing up his night's cases, let alone gotten more than a few minutes' sleep. And now it was click, click, click, click, down the hall of 4ICU for morning rounds.

The first patient, a girl, seemed unconscious as they entered the two-bedded room and Brian Fitzpatrick began reading from her chart. She was small, childlike, but something in her face made her seem old.

"Melanie B——, age fourteen, self-inflicted gunshot wound."

Dead center between her eyes, like a lenten ash mark, there is a purple bruise marking the .22-caliber bullet entry. It tore one optic nerve; she will have surgery to remove the fragments and see if the nerve can be repaired. Melanie may lose the sight of her left eye, though that is not the strangest way to loose half your vision.

When the optic nerves cross at the circle of Willis, they trade bundles. The left optic nerve enters, naturally, carrying visual information from the entire left eye, the right optic nerve from the right eye. But exiting the chiasm, the bundle headed to the left occipital lobe contains information from the right halves of both eyes' visual fields. Headed for the right occipital lobe, a bundle carries all information from the left halves of the eyes' visual fields. That is how a physician can tell whether optic-nerve damage has occurred before or after the optic chiasm. If before, you lose the sight of one eye. If after, you can see out of both eyes, but you only see a visual field half as wide, left or right.

Melanie's damage was before the chiasm.

"How old is she?" Williams asked, "Did you say eighteen?"

"I'm fourteen," she suddenly wailed in a little girl's voice, very softly, repeating, "I'm only fourteen." With her large, shaved head and small face, large eyes bruised purple and swollen shut, she was a baby bird.

Born and raised in nearby Mesa. Mother divorced when she was a baby, remarried and divorced again when she was a toddler. Father still in contact, very much older than mother, in his 70s. You see him in the hallways. "She's a daddy's girl," he told one of the residents, saying that her mother was the harsh disciplinarian but Melanie always got what she wanted from daddy.

Her mother told one of the residents, "Her father's hardly been around. I'm all she's got."

Child has an apparent alcohol problem. She sometimes fought with her mother, even struck her. Threatened to kill herself a year ago. Last week let friends into the house while her mother was working; Melanie says they got her drunk. She was fearful her mother would be angry. So she shot herself. At least that's what her friends said. Melanie cannot remember.

The bullet fragment tore her left optic nerve just ahead of the optic chiasm. A little higher and it would have been in her brain; a little more center and both optic nerves might have been cut at the X of the chiasm; further still, no pituitary gland. A touch higher, a touch farther and a fragment would have caught the major blood-ways to the brain at the circle of Willis or, at the far end, nipped the basilar artery; instant death. Compared to other possibilities, hard as it was to see that way, it was a lucky shot.

Emerging from her room, Bruce Cherny shook his head as they all swarmed down the hall. "Last Christmas they brought a thirteen-year-old boy in through the ER," he said. "He got bad grades on his report card. So he came home, put on a sweatshirt that said, 'Happy Holidays,' put a 38 magnum in his mouth and blew the top of his head all over the wall." His mouth was set. Cherny is short and stocky, strongly built, crewcut, has a tough guy walk and manner except at the bedside. "'Happy Holidays.' Thirteen years old. Do you believe this world?"

And down to happier times, on the Pediatrics ward.

TJ did just as Spetzler had predicted, on June 23, even faster than the Boss had thought possible. Halo brace, leg cast, wheelchair and then walker, he went home. Interviewed and filmed by dozens of journalists, TJ raced up and down for the cameras. A television reporter asked Kerry how she felt. Never given to overstatement, she said, "It's being born a second time."

Volker Sonntag, whose pin had reattached TJ's head to his spine, traced his finger over the latest x-rays the day he left. He would still need to stay in the halo brace for a month or so, but the bone marrow from his hip already was taking root, helping fuse his neck to the occiput bone of the skull. "Is that remarkable? If someone had told me that night in surgery that this boy would not only walk out of here, but would do so a month after Robert said he would, I'd have said they were nuts. Completely nuts."

TJ was an international celebrity. Perhaps nowhere had he so many fans and hopeful pen pals as Germany, where Sonntag, like Spetzler, also was born. The major German news magazine, *Stern*, ran Timmy's photo on the cover in June. Ever since, daily, stacks of mail, gifts and remembrances poured in, sometimes more than a hundred in one day. TJ opened them all.

"Bravo, lieber Timmy! Mach weiter so, sei stark und kaempfe!" Bravo, dear Timmy! Go onward, be brave and fight!

The big computer-printout banner from his Little League team adorned the Mathiases living room wall: "Hang in there, TJ!" Along with postcards, from Germany to New Zealand and across the United States, from the Disney World Mouseketeers, professional athletes, boys and girls and families.

And with his departure, life quieted down again, in a manner of speaking.

Trauma team, to the emergency room. "Okay, okay." Cherny shoved his dinner tray back and headed out. *Trauma team to the*—"I said okay didn't I?" Lose your sense of humor and you're toast.

This trauma call must have been nearby. By the time Cherny got to the trauma room, the rubber-curtained room within the Emergency Department, the chopper was already descending onto the first-floor rooftop in a roar of dust and twigs. He had barely tied on the heavy, lead-lined apron that would protect him from x-rays and pulled on latex gloves when he heard the gurney rolling down the hall, bursting through the curtain.

The young man looked to be about seventeen or eighteen. He had blond hair and a fair complexion. He was strapped to a backboard and immobilized. From the first, he looked like he might have brain injuries. But Keith L——, who was in fact eighteen, had good heartbeat and respiration, intact pupils. As Cherny passed the curved endotrachial pipe through his nose and down his throat, the boy gagged. Gag reflex was very important; if you didn't have that primitive response, chances were your brain stem was shot.

But there was nothing else. Completely unconscious. Knocked out. Not so unusual. According to the paramedics, though, the young man had been found unconscious on the street next to his moped. It was dark, and no one knew how long he had lay there or if he'd been hit or just lost control. There were no traces of alcohol or drugs. Or of consciousness.

The x-rays did not look normal. But it was the CTs that showed disaster brewing. His left and right lateral ventricles were narrow. These huge caverns uppermost and between the cerebral hemispheres drained cerebrospinal fluid down into the third ventricle through an aperture called the foramen of Munro. The swollen brain was squeezing the ventricles shut. It would be important to get a ventriculostomy tube in through the top of his head to drain CSF from the ventricles, or the pressure would destroy his brain. Cherny set to work.

He called his chief backup, and he called the attending neurosurgeon, Tim Harrington. His efforts slowed down the intracranial pressure buildup, but that was all. "His ICPs are near sixty," he told Harrington, who was in charge of neuro-trauma. Not enough blood was getting past the pressure barrier. His brain was starving for oxygen because of the intense intracranial pressure, but no one could find the source of the swelling, it just seemed systemic.

The work was feverish and went on for days, in relays. Now Keith was on a respirator. A man sat by his bedside around the clock. His hair was brown instead of blond, his face heavier, but there was no doubt of their relationship. One evening when Cherny administers the Glasgow test the young man has gone from a 4 to a 3—his pupils had been reactive to light and now were not.

It was time to administer the brain-stem test, to see if, beyond the GCS, there was any measurable brain activity whatsoever. Cherny brushed a Kleenex against Keith's corneas. Nothing. The eyes are the only external organs that have touch receptors only for pain, and if they do not reflexively close on being touched, that is a fatal sign. He has lost his cough and gag reflexes. And now there is one test left. The principal brain-stem reflexes for the ear and eye are adjacent to one another. The result is that if you pour cold water into a person's left ear canal, the eyes should both look to the right, away from the "insult"; if you pour in warm water, the eyes should look left, toward the pleasant sensation. Now there was nothing.

They next went through an intricate procedure, which began with turning off the respirator to see if Keith would begin trying to breathe on his own. Nothing. Finally, they turned the respirator back on, concluding this last test. Now there was only judgment. Harrington talked to the father, who nodded, sat back down, and for the next hour sat holding the young man's hand.

Then they turned off the respirator for the last time.

Cherny confirmed that brain death had occurred at nine twenty-eight in the evening. They presumed that in getting thrown from the motorbike, Keith's head had snapped violently enough to wrench the mushroom cap of cerebrum loose from the midbrain below, at least part way. From that point on death was a matter of time. Autopsy would show the results, and the residents would view them during their weekly trip to Peter Johnson's neuropathology lab.

TUESDAY
JULY
POLICIES/ASSIGNMENTS/SERVICES

DAY	CONFERENCE	TIME	REQU'D ATTENDANCE
1st Tuesday	Morbidity/Mortality	0730	All Residents

MORBIDITY AND MORTALITY CONFERENCE, M&M, is medicine's bottom line. Who got sicker after entering the hospital instead of better? Who died and why? The questions asked are brutally frank and when answers are disputed they are disputed in the most forceful terms. The only doctors permitted at M&M are residents and staff neurosurgeons. No one may record or take notes, and no papers handed out at M&M may be taken from the room.

The crew filed in to the Goldman auditorium, with entrances both in the St. Joseph's wing and from the BNI partnership offices. Francis had had first call last night and he had had no more than a few minutes' sleep here and there as he had to respond to crisis after crisis. He and Cherny sat next to one another so he could pass along advisories about what to expect—what crises had begun during the night that Cherny would have to respond to this morning—and the needed wisecracks of trenchmates. Pager alarms were going off at a higher than normal rate through the auditorium this morning, and they both figured it was just a matter of time before one or both of theirs would summon them, although hospital staff were alerted not to disturb those at M&M except for genuine emergencies.

The first case was presented by Shiu Sing Liu, the only woman resident in neurosurgery at Barrow. Liu was from Indonesia and had originally come aboard on a special fellowship—not a post-residency fellowship—planning to return home within a year or so. But Barrow had arranged to convert the fellowship into a residency, so she would return home as one of her country's few neurosurgeons.

They had never seen an M&M quite like this one and would remember it long after.

Liu presented the case of a severely comatose patient, raising the question of whether his condition warranted leaving him on respirator or weaning him off, to die, based on the various vital signs over various periods from which the neurosurgeon in charge would have to make a decision. The case was presented as though it might have been hypothetical, which M&M cases were not. Now the attending staff neurosurgeons of Barrow voted, whether they would cut off the respirator and leave the patient to "organ harvest" or leave the respirator on, on the slim chance of recovery.

Dr. A recommended continuing the respirator despite the severity of coma. Suddenly Dr. B jumped in and drew an analogy to one of Dr. A's *own recent cases, that of a young mother in fact.*

Dr. B: You recommended turning off her respirator, and in fact she became an organ donor.

The chairs creaked throughout Goldman Auditorium as everyone drew up to close attentiveness.

Dr. A looked around and, perhaps by the sharpness of everyone's attention, saw this had been a setup. The presented case had been carefully drawn to parallel one Dr. A had handled only a few weeks ago.

Dr. A: So you're saying I killed this patient?

Dr. B: (A significantly long pause.) I am saying you made a judgment that, based on this patient's persistent Glasgow Coma Scale reading of 4, she had no chance at an acceptable quality of life, and you advised turning off the respirator.

Dr. A: Yes, I did, and I would again under *those* circumstances.

Dr. B: And I am saying the literature contains many cases in which patients

returned from a coma this profound and long-lasting and went
on to have a good quality of life.

Dr. A: That is false, that is ridiculous! Without severe neurological
impairment? It has not—

Dr. B: I didn't say without neurological impairment, perhaps even severe.
I said a good quality of life. The family made a decision to turn off the
respirator based on certain assurances by you, and those assurances
were not necessarily correct. (Another significant pause.)
In my opinion not correct *at all*. The patient had a chance for
something that you did not tell the family.

Dr. A: That is not true! We're talking about incredible, perpetual,
financially-devastating medical costs here with no appreciable
chance at an acceptable life quality.

Dr. B: It is not up to us, beyond certain limits, to define what is acceptable
quality of life and what is not.

Dr. A: But it *is* up to us not to instill false hope. And to encourage a family
to financially and emotionally destroy themselves in pursuit of
a dream that will not, and cannot, come true is instilling false hope.

On it goes for the better part of an hour. Playing God Himself. Hubris
in the flesh. Is that Dr. A ... or is it Dr. B? Whom would you emulate here.
Think about it, while you have the chance.

If you *can* play God's games, if you have that kind of power whether by
force of will or bad luck, how do you *not play*? Two choices here, 0 and 1,
binary as they come. (0) Turn off the respirator and throw away forever whatever chance exists that a person will emerge from within this hulk, someone
the family had loved and would love again; (1) leave on the respirator and risk
watching a family torn to shreds, every one of them, pouring all their love
(it may require all of it) and all their resources into an icon, a big doll representing a being who no longer dwells there.

Which of these two decisions is not God's?

Peter Raudzens, head of neuroanesthesia, wisecracker, avuncular guide to
residents learning their way through the OR, had begun his medical life as a
surgical resident and he often reflected on these decisions. A small-town boy

from Canada, he had hit the Boston University Hospital full of high hopes, and the traumas of Boston hit back. Day after day, often helpless as a young man or woman died before his hands or was left, despite his best efforts, in a chronic vegetative state. His chief sent him off for six months of research. He loved the research, but when he came back, he knew surgery was not for him.

To know that someone had come into the OR neurologically whole, and, under your care, for whatever reason, had been rendered dead, and then to go on and operate again was something he knew he could not do. But what better pal for those who could?

Francis and Cherny and all the other residents each day were forced to look at death in all the forms and shapes it could come, some well-disguised. But unless they screwed up, they did not make life and death decisions. Yet. They were simply impressed day by day that those decisions would fall to them.

Beyond that, of course, they were being prepared to face something more terrible, iatrogenic morbidity and mortality—treatment-or physician-induced. What you did killed the patient. They had to face that prospect.

Francis and Cherny had first call every third night, the third doctor on call being a county hospital resident doing a rotation in neurosurgery.

That meant that Francis, for example, had come in at 5 a.m. yesterday to do the workups on the patients under his care, this month Spetzler's patients, to present their conditions during rounds. After rounds he had rushed off to Sav-A-Day to admit patients who would be operated on today. Then he had visited all the patients again, this time frequently responding to calls from nurses on the floor because there were problems. And every time the "Trauma team to the emergency room" call had come, he had responded. So it went on through the afternoon, when the call came for Spetzler rounds.

Afternoon teaching rounds are mandatory and will be attended by all residents unless they are in the OR. All appropriate radiographs and interesting cases should be pulled for viewing each day. The resident(s) assigned to Dr. Spetzler's service should be present each day for rounds and will make patient rounds after x-ray rounds with Dr. Spetzler, the chief resident [and] the residents on call that day.

As evening wore on, there were fewer and fewer neurosurgeons in-house to handle emergencies, so Francis's pace picked up. Whenever there were problems, he called the more-senior resident on second call, who often called the attending neurosurgeon on call, both of them usually at home.

> The chief resident should be called regarding important ICU admissions, major patient problems, and pertinent issues. If you think about calling, then do it. DO NOT HESITATE.

He had been kept going all night long, spending a total of two hours in the residents' dormitory, a two-bed room off 4 ICU, and what with phone calls and having to leave for floor emergencies and trauma calls, he'd slept a total of less than an hour. Now Cherny took over on first call, but Francis's floor duties would keep him going until almost 7 p.m. today—not as bad as some off-call days. Then he would drive home to his apartment, through Dreamy Draw at sunset. A truly pleasant feeling, and crash until 4 a.m. tomorrow, another off-call day.

Often if someone was sick or on vacation, Francis and Cherny alternated call days, so there were no whole days in the middle.

This was the system, Sonntag had explained, that had come down from Halsted. The tiered system of response and responsibility assured that the junior-most residents got the maximum exposure to every sort of problem they would have to recognize and deal with in their careers. But decision-making, like "restedness," was concentrated at the top.

Sonntag had made it clear that they were the future of neurosurgery. They would see fifteen or twenty years of cases in their six years here. They would begin to operate early and would be permitted to advance as their skills developed, within limits. They were licensed physicians. In their second year, they would be strongly encouraged to take their neurosurgical board exams, even though they could not take those for credit until they had been practicing for two years after residency was completed. Finally, nothing was being asked of them without the purpose of improving patient care and improving their skills as neurosurgeons, and nothing was being asked that had not been asked of those before them.

It was the sort of attitude that brought you smartly to attention. And put the weight of the world on your shoulders even while promising you could hold that weight and more.

WEDNESDAY
OCTOBER

POLICIES/ASSIGNMENTS/SERVICES

DAY	CONFERENCE	TIME	REQU'D ATTENDANCE
Wednesday, except 1st Wednesday	Brain Cutting	0745	All Residents

ONCE EACH MONTH Chief of Neuropathology Peter Johnson oversees brain cuttings, autopsies that are often like black-box mysteries. You look down on the brain and try to guess what went on inside to kill the patient. He begins by reading the physicians' reports on symptoms, on who the patient was, how he or she behaved.

"Patient was a sixty-eight-year-old male, suffered from acute alcoholism and Korsakoff's syndrome. On 1 July began hallucinating that he was back in Germany during the war. Korsakoff's as you know is characterized by recent amnesia combined with confabulation as a reaction to the amnesia."

And all the while he talks, resident Stephen Coons, who soon will be hired on staff, is placing the brain on the large steel autopsy table, while wearing throwaway plastic gloves. It is hard to get used to the fact that this was the patient. Seeing the brain in surgery is one kind of surprise. Seeing the brain as all that's left of the person it once truly was is a new unsettlement. For autopsy, the brain has been fixed in a denaturing solution, the effect on cellular proteins much like frying an egg and solidifying its proteins. The mixture of liquids and brain cells, including both structural cells and neurons, that add up to a fleshy consistency in the living brain, now is solid as cooked egg white and will not break down when sliced.

Korsakoff's syndrome is a product of acute alcoholism. "Recent amnesia" is the acute form of what ails those elderly who have clear memories of distant events and a tougher time with what they had for lunch or were just told. In the acute form there is no recollection of recent events, not even those of two minutes ago. Memory may be relegated to a half-minute in the stream of consciousness, the self spilling constantly forward and unable to reflect. In the face of this void, perhaps in terror of it, perhaps merely in puzzlement, the Korsakoff's sufferer makes up his past as he rambles along, called confabulating. Sometimes there is evidence he knows he is doing so, sometimes not, but he doesn't know what else to do.

"You will notice the atrophy of the cortex, the shrinkage of the gyri." Indeed, this hallmark of both chronic alcoholism and Alzheimer's desease is very evident; what occurred here in the brain is not clear yet, but plainly the cortex is damaged. Think of the cortex as the farm of the brain, the neurons acres and acres of the flowering of the brain, crowded together, sinking their roots into the rich mulch of the fibrous core, a dense multicolored web communicating so intricately that only recently have neuroanatomists like Walle Nauta of MIT succeeded in threading the major communication routes among structures. The cortex is only seven layers deep in neurons. Evolution has forced its shape into the spheroid, the geometric shape that offers maximum surface area in minimum volume. So you get maximum cortical size, for intelligence, and minimum skull size, for strength. Then the seven-layered sheet of the cortex , over time, has folded, and although no one is sure precisely why, the increase in folding as mammals develop evolutionarily indicates that keeping brain volume a minimum while increasing cortical size has something to do with it. The folding results in hills (gyri) and valleys (sulci).

Evolution does not plan such things, of course. It works the other way around. Those lines of creatures who have, for whatever random reasons, grown bigger cortexes and preserved relatively small, hard heads survive at a greater rate than others, pass on their genes more often, and so such brains go onward.

Coons holds the brain in one gloved hand and with his scalpel slices it in half, coronal: a vertical slice from the top following the line a tiara would draw atop the head, down through the brain stem. And there is a hum of interest now. For inside the folds of the cortex there are red splotches of sclerosis, degeneration of the neuronal processes, especially in the Warnicke's speech area. Tough to think straight with a brain like that. The effects of alcohol on the brain, like those of other drugs, are not entirely well understood at the small doses used by the moderate or light drinker. But for those who drink to stupor the effects are fairly clear.

Proteins are the most important structural and functional molecules in living things. Some classes form the skeletons of cells, others the sheets to which cells adhere, others the bricks of cell walls. Other whole classes of proteins do things; all the major cellular activity of the living organism is brought about by catalysts called enzymes. All enzymes are proteins. Alcohol denatures protein; that is, it deactivates it. If the protein is elastic or somewhat fluid, it hardens like the white of an egg on cooking. If the protein makes things happen, the denaturing stops the activity; if the protein inhibits action, the denaturing lets it go on.

Alcohol is one of a small number of chemicals that can get past the blood-brain barrier to affect the neurons themselves. Any psychoactive drug must do the same, and it is generally thought that the simplest mechanism for their doing so is having a chemical structure that in some way mimics compounds the brain already either imports or manufactures.

The brains of Alzheimer's victims look similarly shriveled, as though the hills of the cortex had become narrower and the valleys deeper by erosion, although it's not at all clear what causes it. When the brains of Alzheimer's patients are sliced they also betray within the cortical folds a yellowish stony plaque called amyloid for its starchiness, an accretion of protein-sugar complexes. Looking down at this shriveled, corroded brain, it is impossible not to wonder what whole life evaporated in there, in the trillions of connections of those billions of cells. Brain death is death.

But the death of an elderly alcoholic is easier to take than the mystery that follows.

"Patient Martin H———, male, age three. Boy was perfectly normal until three days ago, when he became lethargic." The onlookers stiffen. The brain is small but looks perfectly normal—except for here, there, where a tiny splotch of red shows on the meninges. Three days ago!

"The lethargy initially seemed to pass, then the mother noticed the boy apparently unable to move his left side. Then the lethargy returned. She brought the boy...."

"Meningitis?" a resident ventures, inflammation of the meninges covering the brain or the spinal cord.

"Obviously," Johnson says. "But that's not all." He takes over the cutting now himself. His face is set but there is a scientific investigator's glow about him as he works deftly. He is a pathologist, and as he slices, he thinks he knows what the answer to this mystery will turn out to be. This section is sagital, straight down from top to bottom, front to back, separating the hemispheres. Revelation indeed. Similar small blotches dot the inside of the brain tissue, angry red marks of irritation.

"Infection throughout," he says in grim triumph. "And it will turn out to be amoebic." The residents look puzzled.

"But that's water-borne," one says, "sometimes found in *intestinal* infection." Another chimes in, "From accidentally swallowing pond water, because it's an intestinal pathogen. Well, from swallowing pond water, whether intentionally or not."

"Or inhaling it," Johnson says. Silence. "This is very, very rare, but not unheard of. If the boy accidentally got the amoeba up his nose, that could have caused the inflammation you see here. It is the inflammation that killed him. And I'm telling you when we culture, we will find the amoeba."

And so they did, days later. The brain, so well protected from the hostile world it paints within its stone-walled, membrane-lined cathedral, has one conduit not completely shut off from the environment, the most primitive sense, going all the way back to the most primitive insects: smell. The left and right olfactory bulbs, sitting above the eye orbits that terminate the optic nerves, are bathed in air. They draw in through their own protective membranes all the molecules of scent. The olfactory nerve is the first cranial nerve. The olfatory bulbs at their tips are the only neuronal sense receptors that directly encounter the outer world. And, however rarely, enounter cells of amoebas and bacilli. The nose is not the only possible tunnel for pathogens to enter the brain—only the most obvious. The ear chambers are sealed by the tympanum, the ear drum. But if the eardrum is broken, infection can enter that way.

Like the other ailments of the brain, meningitis offers no clue to cause but refers to effect. It is an inflammation of the three-layered membrane, the "maters" covering the brain, just as meningioma refers to a tumor of that tissue. Meningitis can be caused by physical irritation in surgery, by inflammation brought on by hemorrhage, or like so many membranous inflammations, by virus or bacteria. Meningitis is far from rare, but it is very rare that these disease microbes penetrate the meninges and attack brain tissue itself.

Then it's off at a dead run for another day on call, Paul Francis's turn again. The trauma bells rang three times that morning, but none of the cases turned out to be neurological.

Then, just after noon, the call came that everyone dreaded, one that had come in record number this endless summer. A small boy was brought in, with heartbeat but no respiration, a drowning victim. The Valley had set a national record this year for young drowning victims, usually, like this boy, having fallen into swimming pools by getting through unlocked kitchen or dining room doors. He would be kept on a respirator over night, but there was plainly nothing to be done in this case.

Late afternoon shadows were growing mercifully long. The October sun still is beating the desert into heat-wave Jell-o, this month's hundred-degree days finally breaking all records with more than one hundred since the end of March. Game shows play on every TV, mostly seen by no one; few of the patients in the ICU are conscious by anyone's definition; as soon as they are they'll be moved out to a ward; and the doctors and nurses pay no heed to the television.

Francis is worn, feels battered by the constant rotations of call, the time off barely enough to prepare cases he must present at clinical conference, the articles he must read for Journal Club, when the residents and one or more attendings get together to summarize for one another interesting cases in the major neurosurgical journals.

Like all the residents, Francis defends the harshness of his regimen even while agonizing over it. Here they treat you like a human being, even if you're overworked. Here you see a lot of trauma cases, which is important because that's how you learn to recognize neurological problems when you're the first one to see them; it's different from getting a workup from a neurologist on a referral, when everything's laid out for you and then there are a different set of problems to address. Neurosurgery takes tremendous physical endurance; not power, but endurance. And in your six years here you see twenty years worth of cases, around the clock; it's the only way you can learn.

And Paul himself fought as hard an uphill battle to get himself here as any heard, in a world in which neurosurgeons from the great to the undistinguished have come into their specialty from a surprising number of directions, a dispersal more typical of the ways people arrive in all careers than you would expect for so focused a field.

Paul Francis remembers graduating from Vanderbilt University in Knoxville as his awakening—a very grim one. "There I was, with a thousand other guys, throwing our mortarboards in the air. Some of them were going off to medical school, some to law school, some business school, but they all seemed to have some place to go. I had no place. Why? Because I had been a total goof-off through four years of college. I had terrible grades. And all of a sudden it dawned on me, I had no place to go, and it was all my own doing."

So Francis took the bit between his teeth and resolved that he would go to medical school. "I got a job in a lab at Columbia—not a big job, but in a lab where the director was well known. I worked there for a year, then applied to Columbia Medical School. I got turned down, hard."

On he went, for three more years, more and more possessed by the idea that he would get into medical school; taking courses, working in the lab. "I worked harder at everything than anyone. I figured neuroscience would be the toughest course, so I really went all-out on that, and I loved it." By then he knew he wanted to get into neurosurgery, knew he would have to do better than anyone else, with his vacuous background, to stand a chance. The perfect challenge. He was accepted to New York College of Medicine. His first summer he won a research fellowship to the National Institutes of Health in suburban Washington.

"They loved my work, I loved the work. I was invited back for the next summer. I really felt I was on a roll. Then Reagan folded the program."

Casting about for handholds, Francis heard about research fellowships at Barrow, among other places. He called Volker Sonntag, got the job, and came here, then came again the next summer, and finally chose and was chosen for the long haul of residency.

Ten fifty-five. At the very moment of opening the packaging to do a ventriculostomy on another patient, a call comes that a patient needs to be reintubated: He is choking on his own effluent. Francis runs up the two floors and gets the new tube in just in time—five past eleven—for the three sharp beeps of the trauma bells, and the calm, almost soothing voice that follows:

"Trauma team to the Emergency Room, Trauma team to the Emergency Room."

IN SUN CITY, twenty miles west of Phoenix, four men from the church choir drive to the Schulte home each day and put Jack through his therapy regimen. Shirley is exhausted; she is unsure how she would go on without them, unsure how she will in any event. In July, Jack had taken a turn for the worse. She had taken him back to St. Joe's, not on the neurological service but because he had suffered some kind of spasm. She then had left the room and the attendant with him had just given him his food, not fed him. Jack had choked, and seemed to go further downhill from there. He had remained in the hospital until a few days ago. Now he had a stomach tube for feeding. One of the last things he had said to her, last summer, was a comment on the tube down his throat: Please don't let them do that to me again.

He had been on antibiotics for some sort of systemic infection he'd developed. Now, the only thing he would do on his own each day was to take a handful of raisins and feed the mockingbirds.

Suddenly she realized something she had been denying for months: This was not him at all. In the weeks that followed, Jack becoming less and less able to do, she found she could not eat. Then, one day, tough as she was, Shirley just could not get out of bed. Could not do it.

THURSDAY
JANUARY
POLICIES/ASSIGNMENTS/SERVICES

DAY	CONFERENCE	TIME	REQU'D ATTENDANCE
1st Thursday	Spine	0800	All Residents
Remaining Thursdays	Neurosgy Clinical Conference	0800	All Residents
2nd and 4th Thursdays	Journal Club	1630	All Residents

DR. SPETZLER took the podium as he usually did to begin neurosurgery clinical conference, in which several residents would presents cases and courses of neurosurgical treatment and outcomes, by and large the cheerful conference for a junior resident because, by and large, these were the cases that went right—in which vision was restored, or balance returned, or headaches stopped or agonizing pain went away, or tumors were taken away. But this morning's kickoff was somber, not that they had not known of it in advance.

As you know, Spetzler said, Dr. John Green died two days ago, on January 16. Not only was John Green the first neurosurgeon in the Southwest, but he was the founder of BNI, he continued. Everything Barrow Neurological Institute has become is a testament to his vision and commitment.

John Green's death was not quick and easy. He and wife Georgia went to Paris the summer before on vacation. While in Paris, Green went into diabetic shock, then into a coma and had been rushed to American Hospital there. He had laughed about the episode when he got back, but he was a bit less steady on his feet, his voice a bit less certain. And he was no more likely than he had been to remember to take his insulin.

There was the thing that made the staff people shake their heads. One of the most caring and concerned doctors who ever walked, in feeling for his patients, taking care of them. But if Donna Westby or one of his other secretaries didn't chase him down the hall with his insulin, he'd wind up in a minor crisis somewhere in the hospital. True, he was retired. But the idea of the doctor not taking good care of himself....

By autumn it appeared Green probably had suffered several tiny strokes. They didn't paralyze him or render him speechless, as major strokes would, just increasingly eroded him. He spent his final months in and out of St. Joseph's Hospital. He had one high major high point in those months when the Arizona College of Medicine awarded him and honorary doctorate for his contributions to neuroscience. He died at the age of seventy-four.

After clinical conference the residents split up to begin their assigned chores for the day. Cherny was on first call, and he had a premonition this was going to be a day to remember.

"Hello, Virgil! Are you in there?" Cherny sang out. "You are in the Intensive Care Unit of St. Joseph's Hospital, Phoenix, Arizona. You are looking right at me. Can you hear me? Say hello!"

Nada. Cherny is practically shouting but there is not so much a flicker of response from the man, in his fifties and just out of emergency surgery for a burst aneurysm.

Next he looked in on Audrey M——, 24, suffering from a cyst deep in her brain—deep in terms of how hard it will be for her surgeon to reach in surgery tomorrow, but not in a dangerous place, *per se*, revealing one of the brain's many ironies. The cortex, the surface of the brain, closest to the pia mater, contains virtually all the neuron cell bodies. The thinking-feeling-smelling-seeing-hearing-acting brain is all laid out in a sheet just thick enough to be visible if it could be parted from the rest, crumpled like bed linen into folds and crevasses. The neurons send their output wires and get receiving wires through most of the rest of the brain's thickness.

The brain is a matrix of neurons and support cells for neurons, such as astrocytes and oligodendrocites, both given the generic name glial cells, for glue. Indeed, glial cells form the structural support for the brain's dazzling architecture. The oligodendroglial cells carry out one of the most specialized functions in creation. They put out long processes of the protein myelin, a tough, fibrous thread. The myelin wraps itself around the axons of every neuron, just as wire is wrapped around cable, and they prevent any addition or deletion of electric charge as the charge rolls along the length of the axon. As if that weren't biological wizardry enough, at appropriate spots along very long axons there are breaks in the myelin sheathing. These spots, called the nodes of Ranvier, are sites where electric charge can be given a boost. Diseases like multiple sclerosis result in loss of myelin sheathing. As a result of the loss of sheathing, the brain's ability to control its muscles diminishes as electric charge is dissipated.

Beneath that cortex and its glial scaffolding, down in the midbrain, there are other cortical structures—that is, deeper sheets of cortex that mark the midbrain. These are more primitive structures involved in pure emotion, in organizing memories and in weaving together the complex of images, sounds, smells and other sensations, and time sense, into the structured world we experience.

The lateral ventricles spread out within the upper hemisphere, emptying down into the third ventricle through the foramen of Munro. The third ventricle is surrounded by these midbrain structures.

Audrey's cyst is beginning to dam the third ventricle, bringing on at first severe, then crippling headaches that brought her to neurosurgeon Harold

Rekate. Two nights ago she had a "drop-attack"—a lightning-swift fainting spell that brought her in through the emergency room, then here to 4ICU. She had already been scheduled for elective surgery. Once removed, the flow of CSF will return to normal and she will return to normal.

On to check x-rays when the trauma bells sound. Cherny is down four flights like a shot, ready and waiting as the gurney comes in. The man, in his early thirties, is thrashing and screaming obscenities, a remarkably ordinary reaction to pain or trauma in totally unconscious men. Cherny, two nurses and the trauma surgeon are holding the man down while he gets strapped in. "He damn well better not have a neck injury," Cherny says.

"He's seizing!" a nurse yells. "Get 5 milligrams of valium." Another nurse unlocks the medicine cabinet to get drugs. The man's nose is bleeding profusely, but Cherny still cannot get the plastic endotrachial tube in. "5 more valium!" Finally the tube is in and blood drains from it.

Larry T—— seizes again. "We're moving," the trauma physician says. "He's down, he's extending. Let's go!" And now Cherny and half the trauma team are rushing the gurney, headed for the CT scan, tubes jangling, the jars on their "trees" being carried along. All they know of him is that he was in a one-car rollover on the highway. He has few visible wounds: black eye, banged knees.

On the CT, at the level of the pituitary—at the circle of Willis—they see blood in both temporal lobes that sit armlike tucked into the side of the parietal and frontal lobes. They rush him to the operating room. Cherny has called Rekate, who is on call and on his way in. Cherny leaves Larry, paralyzed by drugs, with the chief residents. Cherny already had three pages in the time it took to get the gurney up here to the CT scanner. And now, before he can answer them, comes softly, "Trauma team, to the Emergency Room —"

One page is from 4 ICU so he answers it—a medication adjustment question that takes ten seconds to answer—then he calls the second page from the nurses station. A thirty-three-year-old man in the mountain mining town of Globe has begun having seizures after two free years and— Bring him in, Cherny says. Page three: Mr. M——'s shunt has begun malfunctioning postop for an aneurysm. Since CSF is not being properly shunted and brain tissue is still swollen from surgery, the intracranial pressure is building up. They are sending him from 6 East down to the Emergency

Room. "Perfect," Cherny says. "I was just headed that way."

He is in the trauma room when they bring in the medevac from White River, an Apache Indian Reservation. He had been fine after treatment for a pre-existing medical problem, then had collapsed. The Indian Health Service clinic thought x-rays showed a skull-base fracture. Cherny ordered the man taken to CT scanning. Out in a patient room in the Emergency Department he finds Mr. M—— unconscious and moaning, nurse at his side, and he checks the intracranial pressure. It's high.

Residents often install ventricular bolts or tubes in the top of the skull to drain CSF. But installing a shunt is a surgical procedure. The thin shunt tube is brought out of the skull top and run under the scalp, down the neck and, usually, into the abdominal cavity, where it permanently drains excess CSF. So he called Harrington, the second-call attending, and now Harrington was on his way in.

Trauma team— "I'm already here!" Cherny said. A young man, late teens, arms splayed down the side of the gurney. "He has gag, that's all." Not much. "Self-inflicted gunshot wound" to the right temple. Blood trickles from his left ear. A tiny dark bullet hole, and surrounding it the perfectly circular burn of the muzzle. Police at the scene covered his hands with plastic bags to hold any powder-burn residue there, to indicate if the wound indeed had been self-inflicted.

His name is John B——, and in his pocket is a Dear John letter, in the traditional sense of the phrase. The letter seems conciliatory, but who knows?

Back to Larry now, the earlier rollover. His sister is here, crying. Cherny speaks to her gently in the waiting room off 4ICU. "The risks of surgery are death, paralysis and infection," he says. "But I'd say his risks from all those are less than two percent. The risk without neurosurgery is certain death."

"But he still could die, even with surgery?"

"Yes."

"I'll call our mom and dad. Could he be normal?"

"Yes."

"I have to tell you. He doesn't talk to us much. He's a compulsive liar. He told us he had laser surgery last week. But he's always done that, to play on our sympathy. We can never tell. But you might need to know that."

"Thank you. As for prior surgery, yes—" he pauses to consider his next words but the beat is picked up perfectly by: bong bong bong. *Trauma team*—

It is now 1:05 a.m. Two neurosurgery suites are operating. And they will go on all night. The gunshot wound turns out to be the result of Russian Roulette; there were witnesses. Rekate notes that John B—— performed a perfect prefrontal lobotomy on himself. The White River man had a seizure while standing on a ladder and fell off backwards, smacking the back of his head and giving himself two subdural hemorrhages. These are less serious than subarachnoid; the bleeding is within the dura, so pressure-relief is important; but blood is not damaging brain tissue, as it would be beneath the lower arachnoid mater.

The next trauma call was a Flagstaff man with a malfunctioning shunt, almost the twin of the case now on the floor.

Cherny will not sit again tonight, let alone sleep. He will wash his face and hands in the morning, just in time for rounds.

JACK SCHULTE WOUND UP at Boswell Memorial Hospital in Sun City, where he had started out nearly a year ago. Shirley had called her kids last October, when things got so bad. Within six hours they had taken time off from their jobs and were on their way to her. They got her a round-trip plane ticket to Cincinnati and they brought her back, in more ways than one. That was the kind of family they were. Shirley had put Jack in a nursing home while she was gone. But when she got back home a month later, Jack took a turn for the worse and had to be hospitalized. He now had a massive, systemic infection that the doctors could do nothing about. His blood had thinned out till it was water, one doctor told her.

On March 19, he died. Now, even just a few days later, she was trying to tell herself that he had truly died April 24 the year before, as he cut that fallen saguaro. She remembered and loved that man wonderfully, deeply. That was the day to remember, not all the days she tried to fill for what she imagined was going on inside, that may or may not have been. Although she could not put much into words so soon, she would begin pulling together. And much later, still far from done putting her life together, she would have this much perspective on the terrible ordeal:

The operation was the only chance Jack had, so it was not the wrong decision.

Jack did not suffer. He did not die in pain.

She blamed herself for not being more constantly by his side. She had to stop doing that.

Her neighbors in Sun City had proved to be the best friends she'd ever had in her life, long after she thought she would make such close friends.

She was singing again, putting together the Easter program of "Hallelujah," Jack's favorite piece. She had been invited to sing at a wedding in spring. That was entirely the right idea.

She had traded in her boat of a car and bought a Thunderbird, just as she'd ribbed her mother for doing when she had become widowed.

All in all, as she summed things up, it's better to die on the golf course.

FRIDAY
MARCH
POLICIES/ASSIGNMENTS/SERVICES

DAY	CONFERENCE	TIME	REQ'D ATTENDANCE
Friday	Sonntag Rounds	0645	All Residents
	Neuropathology/ Neuroradiology Conference	0730	All Residents
	Grand Rounds	0830	All Residents

VOLKER SONNTAG, vice director of Barrow Neurological Institute and spine specialist, supervised the residency program. Sonntag rounds tended to be more fun than others, thank God, since they took place over breakfast when the first-call resident had likely not been to bed yet and everyone was hoping to make it through the last regular week day. More fun, though, not because of the subject matter, but because of the man running the show.

Sonntag ran whatever he could like a show, with a boffo sense of humor and a thick German accent that seemed made to tell a joke. He and his brothers and mother had fled eastern Germany at the close of the war, settling in the then-small town of Phoenix not long after John Green had gotten here. Their existence was barely middle class. The brothers worked through the scorching summers on chicken farms. Sonntag worked his way through Arizona State University as night manager of a Jack in the Box. He graduated in the University of Arizona's first medical school class in 1971 and then went to Boston for residency with Bennett Stein, while he was still at Tufts.

Spetzler and Sonntag were a study in contrasts. The Boss was the picture of concentration and calm, no matter what went wrong in the OR. Then he would take off on wild glacier-skiing trips or other hair-raising adventures to break the strain. Sonntag would more likely finish up a surgery by breaking into a cracked-voice version of an operatic high C. He would be cracking jokes in Sonntag rounds, in between perfectly serious instruction. He took his laughs when he could get them. Even though he and Spetzler were the same age, there was something in him of your father's younger brother, who would roughhouse and fool with you while the old man was telling you to be serious. One morning, for example, Sonntag was seen walking up the drive off Third Avenue toward the office, suit and tie, briefcase, the mien of a serious neurosurgeon, when he looked down and saw, as though for the first time, the horizontal beam marking the parking lot's edge. He stepped up onto the beam and, hands outstretched, walked its length; glanced about for observers, then continued his march to work.

It is Sonntag who introduces the new residents to the Glasgow Coma Scale with a new level of seriousness. They learned of it in medical school, probably used it in their first year internships. Now they would put it together in a chain of neurological tests to help them understand what was going on "in there" by just looking at what was happening out here. This morning Sonntag would go over reflex responses that would tell you what peripheral nerves might be damaged. In some ways Sonntag rounds were the perfect complement to Spetzler rounds. Spetzler took them inside, with angiograms, CTs and MRIs. Sonntag's interest in the spine, just the long tail of mammalian brain extension, made his focus naturally on the outward behavior that indicated inner trouble.

For example, as he explained today, certain reflex reaction to stroking the bottom of the foot with the speculum would indicate brain-stem damage. But, now look, this next type of reaction would indicate damage much farther down the spinal cord, at the level of L2, the spinal cord being measured off according to its numbered vertebrae, from C1 at the neck (cervix) juncture with the skull down to the Ts of the thoracic region and concluding with the Ls of the lumbar spine. Just as an organizer of motor response, the brain is incredibly sophisticated and subtle.

For example, the entire cortex is divided into functional units, so strictly territorial that one discreet little neighborhood of the cerebral surface receives sensation from the foot, and its adjacent neighborhood gets it from the knee, and so forth, right on to the tongue's area of the sensory cortex being surrounded by that for the mouth on one side and throat on the other. Wilder Penfield created what has been called the homunculus, a drawing of the body spread across the areas of sensory cortex onto which each body part is mapped. Likewise, stimulation of adjacent areas of the motor cortex, found atop the brain just opposite the sensory, causes movement in neighboring body parts, and Penfield drew a similar homunculus for the body mapped onto the motor cortex.

And if you know how to read just right—always emphasizing the importance of the eyes as a purveyor of information from within, Sonntag says—you can know what you're looking for if and when you decide that scans must be ordered.

Now flip Friday around. Lunch is over. Admits are done. Time for Spetzler rounds.

If you had a particular type of brain image called a PET scan that highlights brain metabolism, showing where the brain is burning lots of glucose at any given moment, and you knew what activity a person was engaged in, you could tell what part of the brain was engaged. So if you were running, you would expect to see bright light along the edge of the motor cortex stimulating the legs, perhaps with concomitant activity in the sensory cortex if you were getting tired and your legs hurt. And if you were talking, there, the mouth-control region would be moving. But not only the motor strip would light up. The regions of the brain involved in speech would also be burning brightly.

Now consider reading, which you are doing now. You'd see the occipital lobes, at the back of your head, glow as this story pours in through your eyeballs and down the optic nerves. But then you'd see the auditory area in the temporal lobes, just over the ear, and speech areas a bit higher and both fore and aft light up, because what you are doing is an analogue of listening to speech. People normally learn language orally and aurally long before they learn to read.

Now picture all that in your mind's eye, your brain glowing with activity in each separate region. The wonder is, you *can*. How did your brain learn to make all those connections? After the basic architecture was laid down by the time of birth, how did your brain get wired, or re-wired, to make such different functional regions hum together over these black symbols on a white page?

Learning in the brain obviously results in structural changes, architectural changes. Not so odd when such "learning" is being done in a plant as it reaches upward to the sun, reacting in ways that keep its leaves pointed sunward. And not so much surprise in the reflexes of the Pavlovian dog, whose brain wiring is altered—whether by a moved neuron wire or changed chemical flow—so it drools at the sound of a bell as it once did only for food. But stop and think where such simple things end.

Think how our brains must be *physical* creations of the world they witness, as well as of the inherited program. Perhaps one theme in the cerebrum of those two residents over there is the result of patterns of neurons firing that resulted from early hearing of scripture preached, or from singing, or discovering Socrates, just to strike the positive chords. Maybe thousands of other themes are the work of thousands of other architects of the three-pound world behind our eyes, working at a distance of thousands of years or working right now, but working at a mind-boggling distance—from outside. No hands. No wires. The brain is a creation of other minds. Or is it that the mind is a creation of other brains?

Watch these blue-gowned residents clustered around the glowing wall in Radiology as Robert Spetzler goes over first one view of brains, then another view, then another. These views were obtained by means of some of the most complex constructions the mind has ever toyed with, both in terms of the theory behind why they work and the demands and tolerances of the machines.

Why would anyone believe that an angiogram and MRI and CT scans all represent different projections of the brain of Jennifer Turner? More importantly, why would anyone believe there are analogies between these images and what they would see if they were really looking at her living brain?

Their imaginations were schooled, and are being schooled right now, so that in the future they will be a notch richer in seeing the filigree of blood vessels, a tad corrected envisioning the coronal plane, finer in focus, and at last an order of magnitude profounder in connections perceived. Six years later, the residents will not see the same.

They literally put their heads together, not touching-close but they all lean in a bit as he talks, prefacing his talk, as he often does, by twisting his surgical cap askew. It may be that as this process occurs over six long years you could trace the growth of new axon connections in their brains; that pre-existing filaments from certain brain cells now will have many more spidery root-hairs up against them in synapse, their *boutons* like lips pressed within an angel-hair of the axon's surface to receive neurotransmitters.

Maybe. But sure as they stand here in a darkened room over Phoenix, Arizona on an April evening, this is a meeting of minds. The brain is an invention of the mind, and they are here re-inventing it.

They are looking at Jennifer Turner's angiogram, left lateral view, a collection of wormlike lightnesses rolling like tumbleweed out of the dark. They see a brain with an aneurysm ready to blow, too far down to have a prayer of reaching it.

But they did reach it. Remember that. They had made a difference.

"I'm getting out of here," she had told them. And she did, three weeks post-op, fit as a fiddle. She still had a slight double vision that the doctors said was residual irritation of the oculomotor nerve but should clear up. It did. She went back to work, although making less money than before because she still couldn't work full time.

She lives in a trailer of her own, shares it with Marc Anthony, an honor-roll student in the sixth grade now, and her boyfriend, who is out with a buddy hunting in the desert. "I've always thought of myself as a good Christian woman," she says. "Life just got out of hand, but everything is okay now."

Initially she found the local scene a little tough to get back into. Many of her friends were still using drugs or drinking too much. "They hadn't been scared straight like me."

Bills have been a problem. The cost of her stay at St. Joe's: $58,770.89. Although she was covered by her then-husband's military health insurance, the government has been trying to recover at least some of the money from her.

Her hair is longer again, though not as long as it had been. She has a light-up-the-room smile and a pretty face, though she's gained some weight and is annoyed at that. "That's one thing the crystal did," she says, "Not that I'd ever try that again. My life is good now. Marc Anthony is just my treasure and my boyfriend works too hard, but he's great."

Remembering back to the night she was brought in to St. Joe's, the low point of her life, she says, "First, the most scary thing is that whatever this is, that's happening inside you, it's out of your control. The scary thing is that you're not in control at all. And then the doctors take control. And then when Dr. Zabramski told me what they were going to do, it was the end of the road. It was like I wasn't even a person anymore, that nothing I could do or say meant anything or mattered to anyone. I had already stopped being a person."

She says, "It seemed like the one thing I still had that was mine was my hair." She laughs with complete merriment at herself. "Aren't women something? *I couldn't let them cut my hair.* Can you imagine, trying to perform brain surgery on somebody without cutting their hair?"

"COME UP TO MY ROOM," TJ says eagerly. "You have to see all the things I got." His father, like clockwork, is upset: "TJ, be careful on the stairs! Use your cane, you're going to fall and hurt yourself!"

He has to show off the hole his halo brace made in the wall, the time he did fall. His proudest gift: Grand Prix race driver Eddie Cheever's helmet. Cheever took third place in the first Phoenix Grand Prix in June. Posters from the Phoenix Suns basketball team—the Suns' gorilla came to TJ's going home party, along with a dozen crew members from TV stations, reporters and photographers—and the Cardinals football team. An invitation to be a guest of the Phoenix Firebirds minor league baseball team; he's especially looking forward to that. Remembrances from the Air Force Thunderbirds, Tommy Lasorda, the governor of Arizona (an autographed baseball) and the mayor of Phoenix (the same.)

The biggest gift so far: A cruise from Norwegian Lines for the whole family from Miami to St. Thomas in the Virgin Islands, as soon as Timmy is medically fit. But there is a painful irony in the inundation of gifts and remembrances: The family is buried under bills. Kerry and Bob Jackson clean vacant apartments in return for their own rent, while Tim looks for work. The Phoenix economy is in a bad slump.

The bill for TJ's surgery and treatment at St. Joe's: $130,000.

Because of Mercy Care, the sisters' charitable program for patients who cannot pay, and the state's health care plan for the indigent, the family does not have to pay any of this. But Tim worries about where a job will come from. He broods a lot.

"I've never had to take aid to dependent children or anything like that," he says. By the end of July, they'd just gotten their first food stamps in the mail, and he had applied for unemployment.

And there is TJ to worry about. "He's always attempting too much, too soon," Kerry says. "He always has."

TJ is anxious to begin fifth grade. He likes math best of his school subjects, but what he really wants to be when he grows up is a professional baseball player. "I don't know if I can," he says. It is the only time he has looked older and wistful.

For a little while longer, TJ would be wearing a plastic neck collar. Adults with simple whiplash are sometimes stuck in such for half a year or better. Sonntag removed TJ's halo on July 25, three months from the accident, less a day. The halo had left a toll, however transient. The skin on his chest and back dried and itched under the leather vest, and his head was agonizingly sore when the pins of the halo came out—though he boasted of swimming the width of the apartment complex pool under water *in* the halo brace. "I can only swim under water because I can't turn my head," he explained.

He had gotten a new bike for Christmas. But there was a touch of sadness about him, mixed in with all the joy of restored life. He had spent six conscious weeks at St. Joe's as a prince, whose every move and bit of mischief was a pleasure, an affirmation of life. He would go off to be a kid again, like other kids. Have a struggle in school. Get his skateboard stolen. Interviewed by a local newspaper reporter on the first anniversary of his surgery, he had boasted to her how he had climbed a tree and fallen out. But he hadn't hurt himself a bit. Elfin grin. On and on.

Fugue

HASSAN AND SALEM EL REFAI kicked at a soccer ball, squealing with the delight of three-year-olds engaged in their favorite sport, each tugging at the other, alternately pulling and being pulled. Spetzler watched attentively, awed by their agility. They ran and played like normal boys, yet they were anything but normal. They were one in a million longshots of nature, and eventually what made them different would kill them, without radical intervention.

Onlookers that April afternoon in Barrow's Magnetic Resonance Imaging suite saw Siamese-twin boys, joined at the crowns of their heads, as they roughhoused while arrangements were being made to image their brains. They saw a startling and engaging series of acrobatics. The boys carried themselves with heads bent at nearly right angles, a fringe of curly brown hair encircling their common crown; they moved with ease and quickness, their bodies having steadily developed from birth to meet the unique challenge of their skull formation.

The brain images Spetzler examined with colleague Wolfgang Koos that day were equally startling. They saw glowing images of two brains inside a single, tubular skull, their tops grown pressed into each other so tightly that they met in a flat plane, the spheroid contorted to a cylinder, yet grown so naturally that the boys suffered no neurological impairment whatsoever. That made this afternoon's decision all the more dramatic, but no less revocable: It was time to separate them.

The saga of the boys' odyssey from a poor village in Libya to Vienna's university hospital to Barrow was a parable of progress. Each facet seemed invented to illustrate the fruits of increasing international communication, or a new power of resolution of what the eye could discriminate, or a leap forward enabled by technology but carried out with hands that had to rehearse endlessly to learn their new, ever-more-intricate routines.

Maybe all that was true of every major case, for in many ways each was the one for which you had trained all your life and each was the one for which all the technology brought to bear had been invented. What else *was* a major case?

The twins had been brought here by Learjet from Vienna because BNI had a new means of angiography, the imaging of blood vessels, that had none of the hazards of the traditional methods and added new benefits. The Magnetic Resonance Angiography developed here by Paul Keller, Barrow's Ph.D. physicist, would enable the neurosurgical team to see the blood vessels the boys shared with a fineness never before possible, and that would be the key to attempting this separation. Keller was one of a handful of scientists around the country bringing imaging to such high resolution that the pictures of brain structures available plainly showed structures in living brains that a year earlier had been visible only under a microscope, and did so without invasive techniques. Ordinary angiography required the injection of a high-contrast dye to make the vascular system stand out, and many patients had reactions to the dye—even, rarely, fatal ones.

MRI is based on the principle that molecules and their component particles vibrate with their own signature frequency, called the magnetic resonance. The giant donut of an MRI looks like a CT scanner and is just as dependent on the computer to draw pictures based on the data it receives in scanning. The data in this case are all the locations and concentrations of protons, which are hydrogen molecules stripped of their electron. Water is very high in hydrogen concentration. Going from these basic principles to images that appear photographic is a saga all by itself.

Spetzler was a true admirer of new technology, and the new scanner showed why. Tools set the limit of what you could achieve; tools determined the clarity with which you could see. Neurosurgeons must know where they are going to within a hair's breadth, a knowing they develop by watching their mentors operate, looking at scans, looking back to the living brain, back to the scans. But Spetzler and Koos would have to get all their understanding from these images alone, because no one else on earth had cerebral blood vessels like Hassan and Salem. And they would have to understand the boys' unique brain vascularization perfectly before they operated in order to plan out in minute detail what they would do and when they would do it, choreography of a performance that would cover sixty hours over ten days. And they would have to beat the worst odds. It had never been done before successfully in a case anywhere near this complex.

Siamese twins occur only once in 100,000 births. Those joined at the head are rarest of all, occurring fewer than once in a million births. Nearly all such "craniopagus" twins quickly die. A few had been separated right after birth, and one or both generally died. One or two lived on as perpetual medical emergencies, or lived only by some dubious definition of life. South African surgeons performed the first truly successful operations on head-joined twins, but they were linked only at a small area in back of their heads, and there were no shared internal structures.

Identical twins occur when a single fertilized egg splits once in its entirety instead of immediately beginning the steps leading toward differentiation, steps which ultimately will yield the trillion or so highly specialized cells of the newborn. Siamese twins are produced when that split is incomplete. The partly divided cells continue sharing common structure, and what that structure is destined to become determines where the twins will be joined.

Probably the most remarkable case of craniopagus twins in history occurred in India early in the nineteenth century; a normal-looking boy was born with a twin's head fused upside down atop his own at the crown. But the "twin" structure ended at the neck, a fleshy bulb. The fragmentary twin reacted to light, sometimes looked around and attempted to nurse—all reflex actions. The twins were displayed as freaks by their impoverished parents, until they died at age four of a cobra bite.

Salem and Hassan were able to survive birth because of two of the brain's most remarkable properties: plasticity and the unique method by which vascularization occurs. The brain can be deformed to enormous degrees, if the deformation is done very slowly. And arteries and veins are sent into and out of developing tissue in response to the tissues' demand for oxygen. A clump of cells sends out a messenger called angiogenesis factor, which draws developing blood vessels to the cells like a plant shoot to sunlight.

The boys had normal cerebral arteries to pump their brains a constant, oxygen-rich blood supply. But once blood has dropped its oxygen, it must be sped out of the brain by the venous drainage system, microscopic filaments feeding into larger rivulets of veins, in turn emptying into the major drains, and this drainage must not be interrupted. Oxygen-depleted blood's backing up in the brain is as dangerous as its not getting there; either eventually will prove fatal.

Among the most critical and the largest cerebral drains is the vein called the sagittal sinus. It runs like an arrow straight down the brain's center, front to back, collecting blood from both hemispheres, draining directly into the giant jugular vein that drops straight to the heart. Hassan and Salem did not have a sagittal sinus.

Their developing embryos made a life-saving adaptation as their brains increasingly pressed together. A vein as large as the sagittal sinus formed in a ring around the circumference of their brains. All the subsidiary veins in each boy that would have poured into the sagittal sinus fed into this ring. Normally, the left and right hemispheres send blood to the roof of the brain to empty from the left and the right into a single, long pipe. Now, each boy's left and right hemispheres sent the blood upward into the common circle. At the back of the boys' brains, looking like a tie in a loop of string, two veins branched off, one heading "south" toward Salem's jugular, the other "north" toward Hassan's.

In order to separate the boys, Spetzler and Koos would have to split the ring, allotting half to each twin. That would mean cutting off half of each boy's veins draining into the ring. That was what other doctors said no one could survive.

How could it be survived? Only possibly in this way: Like traffic flowing along a major thoroughfare that is suddenly blocked, blood encountering a closed vein will seek an alternate route. Major brain areas always have multiple veins draining them. That makes loss of a vein survivable, though extremely dangerous. Cars jamming an alternate route back up; blood doing so causes the alternate vein to swell before the drainage backs up. The swelling itself can be fatal, but if it occurs gently enough, gradually enough, the brain may accommodate itself to the new system. Ultimately blood has to resume draining at normal speed for life to go on. The scheme was as meticulous and painstaking as it was bold: Solomon-like, they would now have to decide for each of dozens of veins that *this vein will go to Hassan*, and *this vein will go to Salem*, step by step around the ring. And step by step around the clock, down the days of more than a week.

And step by step they would rehearse it, together and apart, through three months. What was the quality that such repetition of procedure brought to the performance? Precision, the direct physical analogue of resolution in vision. Why does the musician rehearse the same measures, the gymnast repeat the same pieces of a complex performance, the basketball player take the same three steps, turn and shoot from just the same spot? To bring ever-finer control over ever-more minute movements that compose the whole.

Practice is the weapon against surprise, the final point of the parable. Now the counterpoint. Bring all the mechanical and human powers you will to the moment of resolution, and everything still will hinge on how you deal with surprise.

"We are like a team," Koos said, "training three years for this." At 60, Koos is a large, powerfully built man with a shock of white hair and a broad, expressive mouth. Koos had been a rising star of European pediatric neurosurgery when he met the young Spetzler, still a medical student but thought of so highly by Paul Bucy that he was sent on a six-month fellowship to Switzerland, to study under Gazi Yasargil, possibly the world's greatest neurosurgeon of his generation.

Yasargil was remembered by many for his explosive fury, his intolerance of error, his dismissal of students, residents, surgeons without remorse. He was remembered as the most controlled human on earth in the operating room, a man who would work for an hour under the intraoperative micro-scope he was developing then, in the late sixties, just to spare a tiny brain structure that even the most caring of other surgeons would sacrifice. He emerged from a Third World village in Turkey to pioneer the most tech-nically difficult, technologically demanding branch of medicine.

And Robert had done well with him, as some did.

In those early, heady days of operating under the microscope, when for the first time one had a prayer of dealing with aneurysms and malformations of the arteries and veins because their tiny perforators could be seen, Koos and Spetzler had collaborated on *A Color Atlas of Micro-Neurosurgery*. It had become a standard around the world. Koos went on to become the head of neurosurgery at the University of Vienna, retaining his specialty in pediatric neurosurgery just as Spetzler had in vascular.

Throughout the years of the Cold War, Austria had asserted its neutrality by maintaining relations with Communist developing countries. From North Korea and China, Libya and the East Bloc, Austrian hospitals had served as a training ground for doctors and Koos had held visiting professorships in their countries. That was how the twins came to him. Born to a poor farm couple who already had eleven children, Hassan and Salem immediately became wards of the Libyan state. Brought from Tripoli to the pediatrics department of the University of Vienna Hospital, Koos had been called in for his neuro-surgical expertise. He provided more than that. Within months, he brought the infants to his new neurosurgical hospital, high atop a hill looking out on the famed Vienna Wood. The twins' father arrived in Vienna soon after. He said that he trusted the surgeon to do what had to be done. If it was the will of Allah, all would go well. If it did not go well, that, then, was the will of Allah. That was the last Koos had seen or heard from the family. He had become like a father to them, his staff their family. They first became the darlings of the hospital, and finally of all Vienna.

But from the first, Koos knew that they would have to be separated. The question was when. Nearly all such twins in the past had been separated immediately; Koos believed that newborns' undeveloped vascular systems made survival impossible. On the other hand, the procedure could not be put off indefinitely. The boys already were developing spinal curvature, the natural response to their having to keep their heads at right angles to move around. Still correctable at age three, by age four it might well be permanent; by adolescence the twisting of their spines would produce excruciating pain, and the pressure on their brain stems probably would kill them.

And from the first Koos knew whom he would need to help him. Spetzler already had an international reputation for carrying out difficult vascular procedures successfully that others would not attempt. So now, in April in Phoenix, the decision: The separation would be done in Vienna, because Koos did not have a license to practice in the United States. Through Spetzler's efforts the university neurosurgical hospital had gotten a Midas Rex high-speed drill and was otherwise well-equipped. It would be done in July. He and Spetzler would put the finishing touches on the second edition of their *Color Atlas*. Spetzler would make presentations of the standstills in London, Japan and the Soviet Union.

And now they would carefully stage the procedure, deciding that on day one, for example, they would simply remove a plate of bone from the front of the boys' skull and snip the ring, cauterizing it. Then they would wait a day to see how the twins' brains reacted to this change in drainage. And so forth. The major effort would come during the second week. Then they would have to make the scrupulously accurate decisions: Is this vein needed more by Salem or more by Hassan?

ROBERT AND NANCY SPETZLER FLEW to Vienna a few days early. Vacations alone together were rare for them, as for most parents. They had put their children, David and Christina, in summer camps of such adventurous promise that the Barrow director felt envious. But now they had three weeks in one of the true romantic capitals of the Old World.

They had met while Robert was a resident; Nancy Baxley was a neurosurgical nurse and they met, she recalled, "over a glioma." She recalls the boy's name, his looks, how he had finally died. They married in 1974, in his second year of residency, so for several years they had little time together. Both shared a love of classical music and Vienna was a great capital for hearing it. A few years earlier, while at an international neurosurgical conference in Japan, they had been reminded of a promise to perform together, Robert on piano and she on the flute, but they didn't have the music with them. Robert had telephoned his secretary, and she had gone to the Spetzler home, dug up the required sheet music and faxed it. They had performed before several hundred people.

Now Nancy would spend her days touring and shopping, their evenings dining and attending musical performances with the Kooses or other members of the neurosurgical staff. For Robert, the disjuncture between days and nights was as usual. He would try to get to bed early to read, get up early enough for the two of them to run a mile or two and do aerobic exercises. He spent Tuesday, July 16 in an all-day planning session with the surgical team, they had an early dinner, and he went to bed early, to dream. The old night before the big case dream.

SPETZLER AND KOOS SCRUBBED in early on Wednesday morning, July 17, and took their places on opposite sides of end-to-end operating tables. The operating room was crowded: assisting neurosurgeons, nurses, anesthesia team, angiogram team, medical photographers. Spetzler's photographer, Pam Smith, commemorated the opening as she would each step, by climbing a ladder and leaning over the scene. "No moving." *Click, click.*

Before:

At the juncture of the twin operating tables lies what appears to be a log of ironwood, dried pale and clean. It is the long, common skull of the twins, shaved of that fringe of curly brown hair. Nearly a foot apart two small faces appear carved into the wood, one facing straight out, one cast slightly downward, both in slumber, perfect cherubim carved into the column that is their shared skull.

Now the faces were taped over with green sheeting, so only the common crown showed, the scalp sterilized in amber Betadene. Spetzler and Koos cut through the front of the scalp, then removed a large, rectangular plate of skull to expose the brains at their juncture. As soon as the surgeons cut through the brains' outer membrane in this first of four planned surgeries, they exposed the single, large, purple vein running the circumference where their brains pressed together. The ring. After all the years seeing it in scans, trying to envision it in reality, there it was. Today they would cut it.

Would the drainage back up, bringing on a crisis? The answer came in late afternoon. Spetzler took up his bipolar cautery, searing the vein, sealing it off. The rest of the team stood by in case of hemorrhaging, anxiously watching and listening to monitors for changes in vital signs. The television monitor displayed the scene through the intraoperative microscope, the cautery looming like giant tongs bearing down on a small thread.

The ring was cut.

"Angio!" Spetzler called for Berndt Richling, the neuroradiologist and an internationally renowned angiographer. Richling had developed a balloon catheter that would enable him to test-seal veins so they could check the intracranial and blood pressures before actually making the cut. Richling moved in quickly for an angiogram. It showed good tolerance. No overall change in drainage had been effected by the day's work; they had simply changed the flow from circular, around the ring, to down the two halves. It had taken fourteen hours for this microstep. Koos, pulling off his operating gown, revealed a tunic soaked in sweat. "It went as expected," he said. The surgeons now replaced and stitched up the bone plate and bandaged the boys. The twins were wheeled back to their room, looking no different than they had fourteen hours earlier, save for a bandage where the fringe of hair had been.

Wednesday bled into Friday. The boys were prepped on the table, the bandage was removed, and now they cut a similar plate from the back of the skull, to split the ring behind, a bit more complex since that was in between the taking-off points for the "north-south" drains. Spetzler and Koos went to work.

Friday's work took ten hours, making a shorter day than the first, shorter than those to come. They cut the ring in the back, as planned, so it was now two half-rings. Again the anxious watching and listening to monitors for warning of life-signs gone awry, again the calls for angiograms to confirm that blood drainage was continuing. Again: vital signs normal. But the outcome so far was really symbolic. Half a ring is now destined for each boy, but both boys' veins were still draining into both ring halves. There had been no need for alternate flow to make up a loss. The team had climbed only the foothills, after twenty-four surgical hours. But there had been no surprises.

Monday. Spetzler and Koos worked some of the day in dentist chairs that allowed them to rest their elbows, but much of the day on their feet, their forearms suspended as they worked, clipping this vein of Salem's, leaving it to Hassan; now clipping this of Hassan's, leaving Salem's alone. Frequently they would stand, twist, roll their shoulders painfully. Another ten hours of surgery and Monday ends.

"We're 80 per cent finished," Spetzler said. "We'll wait a day, to allow the collateral flow to establish itself, and hope there is no serious swelling." The days have been exhausting, but no more than foreseen. And the twins were tolerating each division of the veins far better than the surgeons had dreamed. Onward into Wednesday, probing, cutting veins, separating membrane, though the weight of each decision grew heavier as they worked their way inward, into the center of the brains. Just a short distance in from the rim, the meninges are fused together. That cannot be split in two. Which of the boys gets it? Who needed it most? New membrane would grow back, but until it did, from this moment onward, brain tissue would be exposed to whatever fluid the surgeons bathed it in. Infection would be an increasing threat.

Now it is Wednesday night, 10 p.m., yet surely this day has gone on for days, fusing not into Tuesday but into Monday, one never-ending series of cauteries, angiograms, intraoperative scope moved in, moved out. This is the edge of exhaustion. And now it gets serious. As Richling takes another angiogram, Spetzler and Koos and their team head wearily down down to the small kitchen where Koos has ordered in boxes of pizza. For a long while no words are exchanged. No glances. Everyone stares off into some inner distance.

There is one vein left. One out of dozens, a small vein, less than two millimeters in diameter; nearly all of those successfully cut were far larger. One vein.

They can't get it.

The frustration is palpable. Koos sits on one side of the table, his face buried wearily in his hands, the front of his greens wet with perspiration. Opposite, Spetzler slouches, toying with a piece of pizza, staring up at the ceiling. The boys' brains are swelling dangerously from the trauma of surgery. "To try to separate them with their brains so swollen would be courting disaster," Spetzler says. "With all their transfusions, they're low on blood-clotting factors. A nick and they could bleed to death."

He proposes leaving the boys for as long as six weeks. "Let their brains settle back to normal, let the swelling go down." The blood and fluids will drain. Then they will go back for the final separation.

Between now and then, "If need be, we can go back on an emergency basis to complete the separation," Spetzler said, adding, "One never wants to do these as emergencies."

As though on cue, the boys' vital signs stabilized remarkably well in the night. Thursday morning it seemed clear that the decision to wait had been right. The Spetzlers planned an afternoon shopping trip. Robert took a pager in Koos's office on the sixth floor, but he hardly got it clipped onto his belt.

On the ninth floor the monitors were squealing. Salem's right pupil "blew," or dilated fully, an indication of severe brain swelling. His cerebral blood perfusion fell, blood flow dropping because of a shrinking of the vessels. The swelling meant brain tissues were squeezing down around blood vessels, so blood would need higher than normal pressure to get through; instead there was less. Now his kidneys began to fail. While Salem was losing blood pressure, Hassan had too much; if that continued a blood vessel might burst, bringing on a stroke. *That tiny remaining vein* was draining blood from Salem into Hassan, and no matter how little the drain, it had produced a crisis threatening both their lives.

They began at 5 p.m., Thursday, on what would be the longest and most harrowing day, when they would lose it all, recover, come right up to losing it again. Into the night they worked, Spetzler and Koos on their feet, bent over, much of the time, their hands and arms suspended. The OR was stone silent for hours at a time.

Dr. Stephen Beals arrived from Phoenix. A craniofacial plastic surgeon, it would be his job to split the bone strips that lay next to the operating field, to slice the inside layers from the outside so that he could create new skull bone in enough quantity to cover each boy's brain. Beals and his partner Edward Joganic frequently collaborate with Spetzler, working a sculptor's art on the skull bones to allow the neurosurgeon access to once-forbidden areas of the brain or, as now, to reconstruct a broken or malformed skull. "My God, has it been this quiet all night?" Beals, startled, asked Pam Smith.

10 p.m. Spetzler suddenly leaped back, yanking his hand and scalpel clear. It was a cramp, the first he had ever had performing surgery, caused by the awkwardness of his position.

As midnight passed, they were back in the kitchen, same frieze as a day earlier. But now they had cut through the remaining bone struts. They had passed the point of no return. Spetzler broke the lengthy silence. "Two hours ago I was sure we were a millimeter from the end. Suddenly, there are hills and valleys, cerebellar and occipital poles where they shouldn't be." The expression on his face tells all the meaning you need: Surprise! "There is a plane. It's twisted but there is one plane. Suddenly there are structures in the middle that shouldn't be there, and you can't tell if they're coming down from above [from Hassan] or up from below [from Salem]."

Imagine two disks of clay pressed together, one red, one yellow. Someone presses a thumb into one disk, pressing its clay into the plane of the one beneath it. Then flips the disks and does the same from the other direction. Now if you push a knife between the disks, to separate them, you come to a region where red clay is pushed up into the yellow. Or coming from another direction, there is yellow clay pushing into the red. The trouble here is, it is all brain membrane, and it is all the same color and texture. It would even have the same genetic blueprint, if you could check it: It is all from the tissue of identical twins.

Coming to such an intrusion, which way do you turn the knife, left or right? "There's no way of knowing which way it's coming from," Spetzler says. Guessing would be taking a fifty-fifty chance of destroying one boy's brain tissue; worse, it would be a new fifty-fifty chance at every such encounter. Here of all places, so near the center, so near the end. The nightmare has come true: Spetzler is looking at something he's never seen before, there is no stopping and no turning back, and *there is no way to decide which way to cut.*

Then: "There's one thing left to do," Spetzler says. "We'll abandon going in from that side. I'll come from the other side. Maybe coming in from there, it will be clear which way to do the separation."

This would mean starting over again, from the other side. But the cloud lifted from his face, the decision was made.

Half an hour later, Spetzler abruptly begins working fast, then faster. He is standing, sitting, leaning first to one side then another. Every part of him seems in motion, as though he had hit a vein and must be trying to control bleeding. Then it becomes clear that everything is moving but his hands; his body is contorting around his hands, which move in the same deliberate fashion they have throughout these weeks. "I couldn't see," he said later. "They were beginning to separate, and I had to move all over to see what was happening." Now that he was closing in, he wanted to prevent the worst outcome: that tension between the separate bodies would tear some of the conjoining brain tissue, that now in this final moment, they might bleed to death.

Just before 1:30 a.m., Pam Smith rushed back from the operating table: "They're apart!" With Spetzler and Koos each gently cradling one boy's head, the tables were swung apart, side by side.

The twins were apart.

Beals worked more quickly with a reciprocating saw, shaping skull bone removed from the joint crown so they could literally build a new crown for each of them.

It is after 3 a.m. when Spetzler and Koos scrub out. *"Danke schön, für alles,"* Spetzler said.

Have you faced cases this difficult before?

"Not in terms of the brain structure involved. These brains are unique; no one has ever encountered their structure before. And there were structures, within, where they shouldn't be. No, I have never been through anything like this before."

OCTOBER 16: Pam Smith got a phone call in the Barrow operating room at three o'clock in the afternoon, from a nurse friend in Vienna. It would then be midnight in Vienna, and it occurred to Smith that good news isn't delivered at midnight. She braced herself but after listening for a few seconds began crying anyway. Downstairs, she found Spetzler in the hall outside his office, between surgeries. He probably noticed her eyes were red. "What's wrong?"

"Have you talked to Vienna today?"

"No. I tried to get through but couldn't."

"You better call Vienna." She couldn't say more.

"Why?"

"Please, just call."

"Why?"

"Salem died."

He wheeled and led her into his office. "It was like I'd given him a sucker punch," she said. "He didn't say a word. I went outside and smoked a cigarette. When I came back, he was still just standing in his office, staring. I can tell when he loses a patient it upsets him, any time. But I'd never seen him when he found out. I went over and gave him a hug, more for me than for him. He said, 'What's that for?' I said, 'I just know you did everything you could.' The next day, up in surgery, he gave me a hug and said, 'That was nice of you, what you did yesterday.'"

Salem had died just after noon that Tuesday, less than a week after contracting a lung infection. The surgeries, the transfusions, the skin grafts all had required heavy doses of anti-clotting and anti-rejection drugs, drugs that invariably weaken the immune system and leave patients prey to stray infections. Two days before the three-month anniversary of the first surgery, his heart failed from insufficient oxygen, caused by the lung infection.

Months later, Hassan died. Infection killed him as well.

Autopsy showed that the alternate veins in both boys' cerebral vascular system had taken over and were working well. Swelling had vanished. Their brains were returning to normal.

WHAT DOES RETURN TO NORMAL MEAN? There is no simple answer. Early after the boys' surgery, Spetzler said he expected an "adequate" quality of life to resume, without venturing to further anticipate what that might come to mean. A normal brain carries out functions we can all identify, however ignorant of medicine we might be. A *person* with a normal brain can score 15 on the Glasgow Coma Scale, but more than function emanates from the brain. This is an organ like no other, it has no analogue in tissue or in hardware, often as we try to build analogies to help us understand. A *person* emerges from the brain. How could one anticipate the relationship between the twins who went under the knife conjoined and the adults who might have emerged? How could one have measured recovery if they had recovered?

What makes good neurosurgery? Cushing answered: good outcomes. Whole patients. That seems simple enough but, like everything related to the brain, it is not simple at all. The Jennifer Turners are easy: There she goes, up and out, restored to herself and those she loves. The twins are tragically easy, as it happened. But there is a great gray blur into which many of the "outcomes" go.

Case in point. Spetzler has just received a letter from the husband of a former patient. The woman had had an arteriovenous malformation removed five years earlier, and the outcome had been deemed a success. On leaving the hospital, Spetzler had forecast a complete recovery. The husband had missed a phone call by a BNI staff member doing a follow-up study on post-operative outcomes, so he wrote to tell Spetzler of the outcome. He wrote:

"In the time since this surgery, I would describe ——'s life as very, very sad and depressing. Some would refer to it as a nightmare!" He recounted personality changes, depression, suicide attempts, loss of will, repeated psychiatric attention with no permanent improvement. He concluded, "I certainly don't blame you or anyone else for what her life has become. I am sure she could not have had any better care. Life doesn't always treat us kindly. We need to be thankful to God and caring people for the blessings that we do have. I hope and pray that as time goes by —— will have a more happy and healthy life."

Deeply moved by the man's grief, Spetzler wrote a letter back, saying in part:

"The decisions and the right course for each individual patient are always difficult because percentages become meaningless when you talk about one individual. I can only let you know that we did our very best with ——, that you have my greatest empathy and my prayers that she will do well in the future."

Reputations are built on good outcomes, and if the judgment of outcomes is full of subjective error bars, not to mention unknown consequences, what does that mean to reputation? That's a tricky one, and the subject of much cross-fire in neurosurgery.

Massachusetts General Hospital's Nicholas Zervas says the only way to judge the success of your cases is by long-term follow-up, and the only true success is, "If the patient came in a rocket scientist, did he go home a rocket scientist?" Others say this is unrealistic, that patients undergoing major neurosurgery are usually facing death, not job loss, and therefore there must be a careful articulation of deficit between good and bad outcome. Both Tufts' Shucart and Columbia's Stein point out that Cushing's great success was in preventing outright death. But the 1950s attention was being paid to whether patients suffered permanent paralysis or severe neurological deficits— the type of aphasia, for example, in which all concept of language is gone. Now it seems appropriate to pay attention to lesser deficits, but it would be unrealistic to expect them to vanish, they say.

Then there is another way of looking at outcome. A more personal, subjective and judgmental way, and every neurosurgeon reporting a string of good outcomes when his colleagues have failed faces this judgment. That you are glorifying your outcomes; that you are minimizing known deficits, putting too happy a face on it. Spetzler is accused of that by his critics, and even one or two colleagues who like him say privately that he sometimes exaggerates his results, which are, after all, somewhat subjective.

You can take that two ways: Wilson says it's a ridiculous accusation. Stein doesn't believe it for a minute. They both say it's born of an understandable envy. "Here I sit, a terrific neurosurgeon, and I've had bad results in these cases for years," Stein says. "All of a sudden this upstart comes along and says his results are terrific. It's natural for me to think, 'Sure they are, if you make them look that way.'"

Or you can take it the way Spetzler puts it: "I'm probably guilty to some extent. We all are. We want to believe that things will turn out well. And we want to believe things have turned out well. There is probably a tendency to exaggerate we will never overcome."

SPETZLER THINKS FREQUENTLY ABOUT THE TWINS. "There is nothing worse than losing a patient. It leaves me devastated for days. I am sometimes brought to tears. There is nothing to be done about it. Because you have to take it personally. I always tell the residents that: I don't want to see you toughing it out. I don't want to see you getting it out of your system too quickly. It is a terribly personal thing. Take it personally."

Finally he comes to believe that what went wrong, went wrong years ago. The twins were so heavily and constantly medicated that their systems weakened. The constant new surgeries to repair their skulls contributed. None of that could be avoided by the time they operated. They had intervened maximally. One wants to intervene minimally. What would the minimum have been?

"If this ever occurs again," Spetzler said, "not that it's likely I'll see it, but if it does, I would start much earlier, back at their birth. When they were born, their skulls were soft, elongated as we saw them, but soft. At that time I would put a constriction right around the center of the crown, right where their hair was. Essentially a big rubber band, to keep constant, gentle pressure on the soft skull bone of infants."

And over time, the pressure would pinch the skull-column inward, ever more inward. "And the brain is so plastic, you see, that it would adapt to that growing in of the skull. I don't know, but I think it could work. The brain will adapt to almost any space it's given, given only enough time."

And then, when the twins would reach an age of three or so, perhaps only a disk of a few inches in diameter would remain between them. Without fused meninges, without a ring where a sagittal sinus ought to be. "We would be doing almost minor surgery. That's the important part here. The surgery becomes almost trivial. We let nature work for us. We do the least difficult thing we can do."

20/20 Vision

nine

Robert —
My paternal best wishes as you leave the nest.
Don't slow down until you reach the top.
   —Charles Wilson
      June, 1977

NOT TO WORRY. The Charles Wilson who signed the photo hanging in Spetzler's office looks much the same now, and neither mentor nor pupil has abated in his drive to get to the top, to stay there, or most important of all, to define what the top means in this chairman's career that is half a career.

Academic neurosurgery has three defining elements: operating, teaching and research. Achieving the pinnacle requires major accomplishments in all three. Operating drives Spetzler, as it drives them all. Everything between the opening and the closing, surgery is the thing itself, all the meaning for a surgeon. But surgery is not *sui generis*, a creature of itself alone. You always trained to do your best, Spetzler says. Macewan and Horsley did so, as did Cushing, as did Green. How good your best can be is dependent on the science and technology available in your time— though of course how much you contribute to the advancement of science and technology is an important measure of you.

The tools and techniques of neurosurgery extend the hands and eyes, enabling them to reach beyond their natural limits. Tools increase the power of the best neurosurgeon to resolve a blur into a multiplicity of fine lines, or they increase the power of any neurosurgeon to tackle a problem that formerly had been the province of only the most gifted. Likewise new techniques bring to the cutting edge what had been beyond hope, or they extend to all neurosurgeons powers that had been only for the Spetzlers or Wilsons or Ojemanns. The last, says Boston's Peter Black, represent far more important contributions for a neurosurgeon to make than performing a dazzling procedure beyond everyone else's reach; for ultimately, such new techniques save thousands of lives, turning the cutting edge into the commonplace. A new technique might mean finding a safer route into the brain or finding an improved balance of medications based on a clearer understanding of what was going on inside the brain. Most important, tools and techniques are not invented in the operating room, but in the laboratory.

While still a resident, Spetzler developed a type of shunt for cerebrovascular fluid, to prevent its buildup in the brain, a widely used shunt that bears his name. More recently, he invented a motorized tool to place aneurysm clips. Great physical dexterity is required to place the clips because the long pliers-like clip holder must be squeezed open, then the wrists must precisely rotate the device up to 90 degrees, to align the clip perfectly, all this manual action taking place several inches above the placement point. Spetzler's device uses a motor to rotate the clip to the proper angle and open and close the clip jaws, so the neurosurgeon only has to position it correctly. "It will make any neuro-surgeon a very good neurosurgeon," he says. The fixation with tools and techniques goes hand in hand with neurosurgery. For him, so does an ardent faith in the scientific method.

Spetzler had two defining experiences as a resident. First was the epiphany as he confronted the surprise cerebral hemorrhage, with Wilson at his side but unable to help, marking his arrival as a neurosurgeon. The second is a parable of medical science.

In 1976, Wilson removed a giant arteriovenous malformation in a surgery that Spetzler, then a resident, remembers as spectacular. Such AVMs are clusters of arteries and veins where only single vessels should be, and the high-volume blood flow through their dense thickets prevents proper flow in neighboring, normal arteries, thus gradually robbing the tissues those arteries supply as the AVM grows.

According to what was then the universally-accepted theory of cerebral blood flow, with the AVM removed the patient's blood would finally be restored at proper pressure through the normal arteries. Such giant AVMs were not routinely treated neurosurgically because so many severe complications followed, believed to be a result of the surgeon's inability to remove all the malformation. But Wilson knew he had gotten the entire AVM.

Immediately after closing, the patient's brain began swelling dangerously, and within days she died of a massive stroke. Everyone was devastated, not the least Wilson.

How could such an excellent surgery turn out so badly? Spetzler determined to find out what went wrong by duplicating in the laboratory the conditions that had led to disaster. He developed a theory that ran counter to the prevailing belief. He hypothesized that what were seen as normal arteries neighboring a giant AVM really were anything but normal, for they had undergone radical changes over the years of the AVM's growth to accommodate themselves to this changing world; accommodation is living tissue's common route to survival. Blood rushed preferentially to the massive arteries of the giant AVM, so to get any share these smaller neighboring arteries had to stay maximally dilated, all the time. With the AVM gone, Spetzler believed, they were incapable of constricting to accommodate the sudden rush of available blood, resulting in swelling and hemorrhage.

In the laboratory, Spetzler developed an animal model to test the theory, performing several bypass surgeries on cats, whose cerebral blood flow could be made to mimic that in humans with giant AVMs. He connected one of the animals' internal carotid arteries at the circle of Willis directly into a vein, creating a sudden surge in blood pressure that matched that in the arteries neighboring giant AVMs. Stroke resulted every time. Now, tracing backward through the literature for the fatal outcomes that had been attributed to other causes, Spetzler showed that many had resulted from this misunderstanding of how blood flowed in arteries and veins neighboring giant AVMs.

The research received the top prize from the Congress of Neurological Surgeons in 1976; more importantly, it changed the way patients were treated after surgery for giant AVMs. Now giant AVMs are blocked off in stages, so that increased blood flow in surrounding tissue is gradual; or drugs are administered postoperatively to keep blood pressure low until the neighboring vascular tissue can adjust.

Also importantly, the published research came to the attention of a young medical student named Neil Martin, who admired the elegance of the experiments and the thinking behind them. Martin called Spetzler to learn more of the research and for advice on his own career. Because Spetzler had trained under Wilson, Martin elected to do so, and afterward he became Barrow's first vascular neurosurgery fellow. Martin is now the head of vascular neurosurgery at UCLA, and along with Spetzler and a handful of others, is named by Wilson as one of his great successes. That's the way the system is supposed to work, in never-ending rounds of surgery and teaching and research, each feeding each, the latest knowledge spreading quickly to eager learners, yet surgery driving the whole system. Neurosurgery, like all medicine, has one starting point: *Patient presented with....* An awesome problem comes to your attention, demands solution. And the end is defined by the patient's outcome.

The learners change and become mentors. Each July 1, normally two BNI residents become chiefs, each taking six-month turns leading in administrative versus operating room duties. Fred Williams had now moved on to his assistant professorship at the University of Arizona, Tom Grahm to a fellowship here at BNI, then into private practice in Texas. Conrad Pappas and Shiu Sing Liu followed, supplanted by Hillel Baldwin and Curtis Dickman, who are now running the show. Brian Fitzpatrick and Jay Herman wait in the wings. And the judgment rolls on as well. Whether Spetzler makes good his claim that BNI is among the few at the top of the neurological-institute peak depends on what the residents achieve while here, but to an even greater extent on what kind of mentors they become on leaving. And it depends as well on how sought-after are the next crop of residents who choose to train at BNI.

MONDAY, OCTOBER 7, 1991

The residents marched down the halls in the unvarying morning routine beginning in 4ICU, but there was an unmistakable jocularity in the air. Spetzler, usually so informal in manner, had instructed them at afternoon rounds yesterday that today he wanted "no funny business." He wanted everyone on best behavior. He even wanted a lid on the usual bad-taste OR jokes, the ones the patients never hear. Who was going to hear today?

None other than Charles Wilson. He had come in last night, not, as he had previously, to give the John Green Lecture as a visiting professor, nor on vacation or a social visit. Wilson had come to town for one day just to watch his former pupil perform an arterial bypass, one of the trickiest bits of neurosurgery ever devised. He had come to learn a technique Spetzler had perfected.

The OR was a bit more crowded than usual, but another new piece of technology was being tried out that accommodated more visitors and gave them a better insight into what was going on. The new addition was a three-dimensional television system. Before now, on a big case all the medical visitors crowded behind the neurosurgeon, one by one taking a turn at the surgeon's side to peer through the second binocular lenses of the intraoperative microscope, the only way to see the three-dimensional world. The flat image of the old monitor, like a photo in a textbook, lacked a whole dimension in a world where salvation and disaster are measured in fractions of a millimeter.

Now the world was complete. Wilson spent most of his time with the residents a few yards away from Spetzler, wearing the special glasses familiar to 3-D movie fans, watching the spectacle in full depth on screen.

The opening screen informed that the patient turned eighty last week, gave his name and offered for the record:

STA-PCA BYPASS 80Y/O M

RF SPETZLER MD

BNI 3-D PRODUCTIONS

The first line announced that Spetzler would clip a portion of the superficial temporal artery and feed its blood supply into the posterior cerebral artery, the sort of technique that earns neurosurgeons reputations among other neurosurgeons. The superior temporal artery is an unimportant, one-millimeter filament that provides blood to the scalp, which has many similar sources and can easily do without this one. The STA's major virtue is that it bifurcates into a Y just as the posterior cerebral artery does, is the same size, and lies directly above the critical, deep-brain PCA coming off the circle of Willis. The PCA is deep in the high-value real estate that is Spetzler's home territory. Spetzler's aim was to insert one Y-branch of the scalp artery through an incision in the skull and stitch it end to end with the corresponding Y-branch of the PCA. This would send a new, full blood supply down the PCA into the basilar artery, and out into all the arteries branching off the basilar.

Not only was this bypass technically at the limit of manual dexterity, it was the sort of counter-intuitive procedure that only painstaking laboratory confirmation could bring into the OR. Blood flows up the front of the brain stem in the twin vertebral arteries, combining into the "northern" basilar, with tributaries then branching off the basilar artery laterally in both directions. The patient's vertebrals had so constricted that the basilar was getting less than 10 percent of its normal blood supply. The bypass would send blood "south" from the PCA *into* the basilar—in other words, from the opposite direction. That certainly counters anyone's intuition of a workable fix. But it works.

Given the location, by now the major difficulties are apparent: getting to the posterior cerebral artery, and working down there without disturbing any of the cranial nerves that could begin to spasm just from the brush of a scalpel. But the real trick was not apparent yet, though the real trick was why Wilson is here.

It took a couple of hours to expose and cut the superficial scalp artery, open an incision in the skull to insert this new source of deep brain blood supply, then expose the target. Now Spetzler clamped off the posterior cerebral artery upstream from the point of the new attachment. He used razor sharp scissors to cut one of the PCA's Y branches, leaving it temporarily without blood flow.

Viewing this all, you can see one aspect of the difficulty by matching the dimensions of the instruments as they appear on the monitor with those in the surgeon's hands. What appears on screen to be hedge clippers slicing through garden hose is actually a pair of dollhouse-tiny scissors on long handles. Now Spetzler threaded a barely visible fishhook needle with gossamer thread and, holding the needle in long-neck pliers, threaded through the awaiting sections of scalp artery, pipelines which, out here in the macro-world, looked like thick thread. He leaned over, and over still farther and more awkwardly. Meanwhile, looking back to the monitor, into micro-world, a giant fishhook was threading through the spaghetti-strand of cerebral artery, then back through the scalp-artery segment, now back through the cerebral, until one end of the scalp "hose" was stitched to the PCA tube, one side of each Y now linked.

Wilson stepped in to look over Spetzler's shoulder, then looked back to the monitor. "That's really neat," he said. "Boy, that's neat."

"The tough part," Spetzler said, "is that there's no room to move your wrists." Indeed, Spetzler stood straight over the entrance incision and both his hands pointed straight down, working long-handled grips, one holding the scalp STA segment, the other the needle; he had utterly no leverage to make these fine stitching motions. Wilson and Spetzler talked briefly about possible ways to position the patient on the table in the Mayfield brace that held his head at just the proper angle, and why this one position had to be chosen for proper artery exposure although others would have made hand position much easier.

Spetzler was still threading the tiny scalp artery onto the Y branch in the PCA, and threading again, and drawing tight. Now the end nuzzled down. He removed the clamp. Not a drop of blood oozed from the bypass as blood resumed flowing, now from the scalp, through the skull incision, into a nether region of the brain to re-supply the basilar artery.

The moment recalled an image Wilson had conjured in talking about the most important neurosurgical gifts. "You may have a guy who can thread a cobweb through a shadow, but without the judgment to know when this can be done or whether it should be done, that's not going to work."

This had to be the closest thing imaginable to threading a cobweb through a shadow. But Spetzler is the first to focus on developing judgment and on bringing in all the kinds of support the hands need. The ability to envision in three dimensions has to be nurtured. Tools like the 3-D monitor aid in this nurturing. Better clips, higher speed drills and saws. Scans show you where to go and what to expect when you get there. And the tools of the laboratory tell you what works and what doesn't. Spetzler gets the tools he needs when he needs them from the Sisters of Mercy who run St. Joseph's Hospital.

Wilson no longer thinks Spetzler made a mistake in coming to the middle of the desert to stake his claim on neurosurgery. The mentor says, "He's really turned the place into an incredible show. He's got a great gift for dealing with people and for organization. He couldn't do what he's done at a university. The university would not tolerate a Spetzler. They just wouldn't let one kid get all the marbles."

If you are skillful and lucky enough to get all the marbles, and you know just how to use them, a lot of interesting cases come your way, increasing in number and kind and in the distance traveled to reach you. If you are very focused and totally determined to understand one area of the universe's most complex real estate better than anyone ever did before, then eventually each new case harks back to one before, or to a hard lesson already learned, or to a principle, uncertainly put as you first conceived it, now looming before your eyes as reality rather than abstraction.

He had fused the superficial temporal artery of the scalp to the posterior cerebral artery of the deep brain and saved an eighty-year-old California man for perhaps another decade of life. And he had only shortly before considered the brain's fantastic adaptability in trying to foresee how he might approach craniopagus twins the next time. *The brain is so plastic, you see, that it would adapt to that growing-in of the skull. The brain will adapt to almost any space it's given, given only enough time.* Soon these different lessons would come together.

"Plastic—Tending to build up tissues to restore a lost part.... Capable of being molded," says *Dorland's Medical Dictionary.* Two very different meanings of plasticity in the brain. The first refers to the ability of brain tissue, sometimes in adults and frequently in children, to take up the tasks of brain tissue that has died. Sometimes small children have raging epilepsy that is uncontrollable but is confined to one hemisphere. If that hemisphere is removed, the children often grow up to be completely normal, all the functions that are normally distributed in both hemispheres now handled within one, an awe-inspiring example of neuronal plasticity, first meaning.

And the second meaning, which Spetzler intended in speaking of the twins: able to be shaped and reshaped, able to accommodate to changing conditions. Now came an awe-inspiring example of that second meaning. A string of cases arrived, remarkable for their similarities, though owing less to coincidence than did those cases of that three-years-ago April. These new patients were a mark of Spetzler's growing world reputation, and of the increasing thrust of neurosurgery into the skull-base region that had been forbidden because morbidity and mortality was so high. Now the skull base is increasingly the terrain of the world's top neurosurgeons, the surgeries still on the edge and far from commonplace, still quite spectacular.

Spectacular was the only word to describe the case of Norman Robinson Jr. The boy developed meningitis at the age of eleven; that could have been the beginning, but he recovered with no apparent ill effects except lingering, infrequent headaches. Many if not most children get headaches. Norman was about average in his interest in sports as he entered his teens, but the headaches tended to become severe when he was excited, so he backed off from serious competition. But he was wild about roller coasters, and those never gave him headaches. His father would have preferred a deeper interest in the contact sports like football, rather than the gut-wrenching rides requiring dad for company. Norman Senior was a disability-retired soldier, now postal worker in suburban Maryland; mother Williemae was an Equal Opportunity office worker. Senior had had more than his share of being tossed in the air in tin cans in Vietnam, being flown from one site to another as an enlisted member of a construction battalion. But not to disappoint his son, he took him on the Bear and the Dragon at King's Dominion in nearby Virginia, and on plenty of others on family vacations. Looking back now, he could not believe how lucky the boy had been, year after year rocketing along on roller coasters, going through Gs of pull, his adrenaline rushing, pulse pounding.

The headaches got worse, with no pattern to their onset. Then came fever and, putting the two together, the doctor on the phone told the boy's parents it was almost certainly the flu. But the fever persisted, and on an August Friday night full of thunderstorms, with the roads slick or flooded, Norman took his son to the hospital at Andrews Air Force Base. Now when the doctor said flu, Norman Senior put his foot down. Flu developing for three years or maybe more? He wanted x-rays, and finally he got them. The doctor could not believe what appeared; whether tumor or aneurysm it was too large to be real.

The family was referred to Bethesda Naval Hospital for CTs and MRIs. Now there was no doubt it was an aneurysm, the largest the staff had ever seen. Neurosurgeon Robert Hargraves gave the family a list of the few neurosurgeons in the country who might consider operating on such a deadly time bomb. There were two reasons most would be reluctant to attempt it. First, somehow the massive aneurysm would have to be bypassed, with a new blood supply brought in from elsewhere. The aneurysm occupied virtually the entire middle cerebral artery, coming off the circle of Willis just forward of the posterior cerebral artery. How could such a critical blood supply be substituted? But second was a truly appalling prospect the operator would face.

Hargraves looked down on a bright, lively teenager with a huge smile and a shy, engaging manner. Virtually asymptomatic. Whoever undertook the operation stood a good chance, under his own hand, of leaving the boy dead or vegetative. However life-threatening the lesion—and it beggared belief that it had not already burst—the odds were that the boy would go into surgery whole and come out a disaster. Hargraves had been one of the first vascular fellows at Barrow, and Spetzler's name was first on the short list of possibles he gave the Robinsons.

WEDNESDAY, OCTOBER 23

NORMAN ROBINSON
STA-MCA BYPASS 14Y/O M
RF SPETZLER MD
BNI PRODUCTIONS

What Spetzler confronted as he prepared for the first of two planned surgeries seemed impossible. Cerebral aneurysms commonly bleed or rupture at anywhere from berry- to coin-size. The aneurysm in Norman's head was five inches long and about two inches at its widest, an elongated football.

It had blown up until it occupied one fifth of his cranium. One fifth of the boy's brain had been squeezed back to make room for the aneurysm, with no worse symptoms over the years of its growing than nagging headaches. Spetzler's aim was to do the kind of bypass he had just shown Wilson, but with the added danger that as the aneurysm was uncovered and the pressure over it reduced, it would burst on the operating table.

A balloon that size would likely be instantly fatal on rupture, even on the operating table where the neurosurgeon would have the best chance to control bleeding. How had it grown so large without destroying the brain's ability to function? *Children's brains are so incredibly plastic. Given time, the brain can adapt to any space.* It is as though, because he had said that about the twins, now there had to come a succession of cases to make his point— and to make it in ways he would rather not have it made.

A month earlier, he had operated on a young man named Paul Grasso, who suffered from an apparently-lifelong tumorous growth of blood vessels called a cavernous malformation. The benign growth begins when a single blood-vessel cell grows out of control, into a berry-shaped sack. Invariably the one berry would be followed by others and still others, forming a cluster, rather than the solid mass of a tumor. Eventually, blood would become backed up as the knot grew. Blood speeds up in an AVM; it slows down and clogs in a cavernous malformation. If the blood supply found alternate routes, as had been the case with Paul Grasso, then the growth might not be found for years. In this case, Grasso might have been born with its beginnings twenty-eight years earlier.

When Spetzler removed the growth, he hardly believed what he saw, an infrequent occurrence after fifteen years as a neurosurgeon. The hole within the pons of the brain stem left him looking directly into the fourth ventricle, the lowest and the most remote cavern in the brain. Grasso had a spheroid hole in his brain stem nearly an inch in diameter. And he was recovering remarkably well. Just by growing so slowly over the years, the cavernousmalformation had gently squeezed the pons tissues aside, the problem not becoming acute until the growth began to bleed. Plasticity.

And now Norman Robinson's aneurysm demonstrated plasticity on another order of magnitude, although here it was cerebral brain tissue accommodating itself to its constricted space, not that of the more delicate brain stem. Still, *20 percent of the cranium*. And the final complication—the aneurysm was on the left side, dominant for right-handed people like Norman, controlling speech and other intellectual functions. Spetzler, usually so open to visitors in his OR, today gave out word that he wanted "nobody looking over my shoulder."

There would be no visitors this time. The 3-D television would go unused, but of course they would videotape the entire procedure for residents' rounds and for hospital grand rounds; God willing, even for conference presentations if there might be news to report. They had one new weapon that could help in this case, a piece of technology dubbed the Magic Wand. BNI was one of a half dozen institutes in the country experimenting with it. *The neurosurgeon must know precisely where he is and where he is going at every moment.* The wand would show Spetzler both. The device comprised a computer and a mechanical arm. The computer displayed a three-dimensional image of the head, reassembled from all the patient's CT and MRI scans that were loaded into its memory banks. To this computer was attached the mechanical arm, with a wand at the end of it. Spetzler would place the wand at some reference point on the patient's head—say, the midpoint between the eyes. Then using the computer cursor, he would locate the same spot on the head image on the computer monitor. Each time he matched up a landmark on the patient with its counterpart on the screen, the computer would adjust its reckoning. And finally, as now, Spetzler could simply move the wand over Norman's head and view on the screen the composite scans of what lay beneath, showing whether he was over normal tissue or aneurysm. The area traced across the skull was so large he wanted to disbelieve the instrument, though he knew from all the individual scans that it was close to right on target even in these early days of its field trials.

John Anson, a vascular fellow who had come from Chicago, would assist. They would attempt to bypass the aneurysm and then deflate it, in two separate moves a week apart, to allow the boy's brain to recover in between.

Three weeks after showing Wilson the STA-PCA bypass on a microscopic level, when it was the physical positioning and manipulation of the hands that was so difficult, Spetzler would snip both forks of the bifurcating superficial temporal artery to bring a new blood supply into the similarly branching arteries that fed out of the giant aneurysm.

As soon as they lifted the dura over the left temporal lobe they saw it, pushed all the way up out of the center of the brain. Most of the blood inside the balloon had thrombosed—dried and even crystallized and calcified— and each layer of the hardened blood had pushed the aneurysm out wider to allow room for new blood to flow through the core; that much had shown in the scans. If it was a miracle that the balloon had not ruptured, it was equally a miracle that the thrombosis had not sealed off the passageway, killing the boy with a stroke that would spread everywhere downstream of the middle cerebral artery.

Looking down, Anson saw the internal carotid coming up from the neck, north into the circle of Willis, where it met the anterior cerebral artery on his right. But the middle cerebral artery should have come in from the left. Now the aneurysm erupting out of it had shoved it down to the right, splayed across the middle of the picture. This time, having room to work was no problem. The giant balloon had pushed all the brain tissue well aside and lifted the artery up to their view. In six hours, Spetzler brought in the new blood supply and removed the clip from the STA, and the trickle that had been leaving the middle cerebral artery was supplanted by a normal blood flow.

FRIDAY, NOVEMBER 1

The second day was the devil. That was when they had to drain the aneurysm, routing out the calcification and thrombosis by using an ultrasound probe to break up the mass. That was the day that Anson observed all that could have gone wrong with the slightest mismove. For as Spetzler tugged to bring the deflated aneurysm to the fore, to get a clip around its neck, perforator after perforator emerged from hidden places that had not seemed to be there. Catching or cutting any one of them could have left the boy paralyzed on one side. Looking down through the microscope, the middle cerebral artery loomed so large it filled a fifth of the field. The perforators were like small roots off that tree trunk, an order of magnitude smaller than the artery. Just as Anson thought they were done, Spetzler would tug a little more, and here would come another perforator that had to be gently prodded away from the body of the vessel, so it would not be included in the clip.

And then they were done.

The next morning Norman Robinson began coming out of his barbiturate coma. As was becoming more and more common after Spetzler spectaculars, the news media came. Within two days Norman sat up in bed, shy, beaming at all the fuss being made over him. He was on his feet in days and home in two weeks. And except for having a tough time getting back into the swing of ninth grade after missing several months, it was as though nothing had ever happened. The Barrow team scoured the medical literature, as always. Nothing like this had ever happened before, at least to anyone who lived long enough for a doctor to behold an aneurysm that size in a living brain.

The spectacular cases keep finding Spetzler. As word of a new success gets out, whether at meetings or in the popular media, people desperate for cures, for relief find their way here. He has good hands, good eyes and good judgment, to be sure. Yet each of Spetzler's bypasses involves temporary ischemia, and his growing success in handling aneurysms and other abnormalities of the cerebrovascular system is as much a product of laboratory research as of his increasing finesse in approach, in anticipating what he will see. Interruption of normal blood flow is dangerous; dealing with it requires the knowledge of chemical balances in the brain and their effects. How much can one safely reduce blood demand with barbiturates, so that ischemia will not cause damage? How quickly should normal flow be resumed and under what conditions to avoid vasospasm? This spasming of vessels, which contrains blood flow, is the single most common cause of post-operative neurovascular complication.

Such laboratory insights are important in all neurosurgery, but they are the critical underpinnings of the standstills. As Spetzler had predicted, at this point the standstills had not increased in frequency over the years. They remain a high-risk procedure of neuroanesthesia, refined in laboratory research here by neurosurgeon Joe Zabramski and the neuroanesthesiologists to provide a window of opportunity for surgical rescue. After the year's gap that had preceded Jack Schulte's surgery, the standstills since had proceeded at about four a year, each with its similarities to the others, each with its often incredible idiosyncrasies.

Many of the changes in this procedure have resulted from research coordinated by Zabramski. Directing these efforts has been his major charge since being hired here. His research questions, indeed the research focus at Barrow, revolve around finding new and improved ways to protect brain tissue during interruption of blood flow—cerebral ischemia, whether transitory ischemic activity, stroke, temporary clamping of a vessel during neurosurgery or full standstill. These represent a continuum of dangers to the brain that demand a graduated and shifting response.

Zabramski began work on cerebral protection as Spetzler's resident in Cleveland. "We proved in primates there that barbiturate coma effectively protects the brain," he said. "We extended the work here. The critical part of the lab work is that it helps define the limits of therapies in a way you cannot do on a patient."

He worries over grant proposals and research results, concerns himself with the fine detail of numbers that most of his colleagues abandon for the emotional rush of the operating room. He operates less frequently than the others and then sometimes operating in special suites nearby on a baboon being treated with a new drug to see if it can be brought through stroke successfully.

How has the approach to problems deep in the brain advanced over the years? Consider Jim Youngblood, a living history of the treatment of cerebral ischemia. On a bright spring Friday night in Boise, in the mild belt of Idaho below the snow-covered mountains, he stepped out after work for a few games of pool and a few beers. These had not been Youngblood's best days, in mid-divorce and living alone again, and they were about to take a turn for the worse. He bent down, drew back his pool cue and—pow—lightning struck behind his eyes. Appropriately enough, a thunderclap headache followed. He walked outside, lay down in the parking lot and passed out. Friends who followed saw him go through what looked like an epileptic seizure.

Days later, CT scans showed a buildup of cerebrospinal fluid. Doctors put a shunt into Youngblood's ventricles, passing it out under the scalp, down the neck and into the abdominal cavity where the fluid would be absorbed, the common procedure to relieve intracranial pressure caused by excessive CSF. The shunt would remain there. They believed the seizure had been the result of Youngblood's having been rear-ended in an auto accident a year earlier, and they put him on anti-seizure medication briefly.

Youngblood had actually developed a basilar-tip aneurysm, the balloon swelling out until the countering pressure of brain tissue stopped it. It had bled a little that night. But no one knew that, and if anyone had there would have been little if any treatment available for a lesion so deep within the brain. The year was 1978, and the few standstills involving the brain had been disasters; the procedure had been abandoned.

Just as Norman Robinson Jr. was returning home to Maryland, Youngblood had another of those thunderclap headaches, the first since that night more than thirteen years before. He had trouble focusing on his computer monitor but laid that off along with the headache to craning his neck as he worked. Nevertheless, at his wife Gail's urging, just after New Year's he had a complete neurological workup. He passed with flying colors. No deficits; nothing showing on the CT scans.

But now it was November, 1991 and there were new tools to aid in the search. He had an MRI, and the doctor saw something. It was just a blur, he told Jim, but that was reason to look further. Then an angiogram showed what was either a tumor or an aneurysm. It was hard to know which to fear more. The tumor might be incurable, but Gail, a clinical psychologist, knew the aneurysm could rupture at any time. Jim's neurologist offered a list of five neurosurgeons in the country who might attempt to deal with such a deep lesion. Spetzler's name was at the top.

Jim Youngblood's surgery was a landmark of sorts, in a procedure that Spetzler insists is not marked by milestones. Advances in these procedures, like all those at the very edge of neurosurgery, are measured in small increments. For those interested in tracking numbers, Barrow's twentieth standstill had occurred just as Norman Robinson's father was bundling him to the hospital for x-rays in August. Pamela Reynolds-Najour's basilar aneurysm had developed quickly; she had gotten headaches and fainting spells; in no time she was in the hospital, and in no time out again. She emerged fit and happy, returning to Nashville with her fiancé and parents, who had accompanied her.

The landmark in Youngblood's surgery was that Spetzler gave permission for a network film crew to televise it. CBS had asked him to film a standstill three years earlier, and he had put the network off. Supremely confident or not, he was not sure enough of the procedure or what surprises lay in wait to risk showing a possible disaster on nationwide television, adding a new layer to what would already be profound trauma for a family. Now he gave his okay. The CBS crew had already interviewed the Youngbloods and traveled from Boise to Phoenix with them on the plane. Youngblood's surgery took place on February 20, his 48th birthday—or as Gail called it, his rebirth-day. It became one of Ed Bradley's "Street Stories."

Months later, Youngblood was in fine fettle on the telephone, his sense of humor at full tilt. He still had some numbness on his left side. Though his voice sounded clear, he said, "Folks who've known me a while say I slur my words a little bit, like I've been drinking. I don't drink, and I can't hear it, but that's what they tell me."

Gail said bills for their business had been a problem, worrisome but not insurmountable. "And we get depressed sometimes that everything isn't 100 percent. But, professionally, when I think where he is compared to most people with brain trauma, it's fantastic." Insurance covered all their medical costs, and for one bit of great luck they were very grateful. Jim had been just on the right side of the eligibility timeline for insurance to cover him on their joint policy. The bills from all the physicians and the hospital, she estimated, were around $175,000. Of that, the bills for the operating room doctors accounted for about $20,000.

WHEN SPETZLER TOOK OVER as director of Barrow Neurological Institute, he vowed to bring it to the front rank of American and world leadership in neurological care. That requires top-rank achievements in patient care, education and research. To what extent had he done it? By the early years of the decade, BNI had emerged into the public spotlight with increasing frequency, sometimes often enough that rarely a month passed when it was not the subject of a national or international story. Is this a mark of quality or of "mere" fame? There's no certain answer; separating the glare of publicity from the glow of critical praise is impossible, and there have been plenty of both at Barrow.

But everyone knows the public spotlight is fickle and serious judgment of one's success not to be measured by it. It is by the light of peer appraisal that those in the sciences generally agree to be judged. Accordingly, *U.S. News & World Report* published a special section on "America's Best Hospitals," basing its results on the evaluations of professional health groups. Barrow was named among the top in neurology, a category that included neurosurgery. Months later, *Good Housekeeping* magazine published "The 400 Best Doctors in America," based on evaluations by physicians in each specialty listed. Spetzler was among two dozen in neurosurgery, listed in alphabetical order. And finally, in 1992, the book *The Best Doctors in America* was published, culling the results from extensive surveys of hundreds of U.S. physicians. No less than five BNI physicians were among purportedly the top one percent of American doctors—Spetzler, Sonntag, Rekate, Shapiro and Raudzens.

Proof positive? Anything but, say any number of neurosurgery chairmen who are themselves on the lists. Isn't it strange, for example, that all those neurosurgeons with, as one quipped, "The Good-Housekeeping Seal of Approval," are department chairmen? Wouldn't department heads naturally be the best known among their peers and therefore most likely to make everyone's list?

But the qualms are more fundamental and simpler than survey methodology. Bluntly, would *any* of these neurosurgeons substitute a poll result for his own judgment? Not on his life.

Finally, neurosurgery itself is changing rapidly, its demands constantly shifting, just as Spetzler noted in looking at the past. If it was difficult ten years ago to separate current from past glory, now it is impossible. And how, then, would you begin to estimate potential? More women are entering neurosurgery residencies, though the number is still very small. And more of the men and women seeking matches as they graduate from medical school deliver scientific credentials that are the envy of their mentors.

Looking at the résumés of candidates applying to Barrow each year, Spetzler says, "It's quite shocking to realize that with the credentials I had coming out of medical school, which I thought were fairly impressive, I now could not be admitted into my own program."

A subtle compliment on the quality of BNI's applicants? Partly, but his look is dead serious and there is an edge in his voice by now quite familiar. There

may be an end to neurosurgeons, but there will be no end to their competitiveness. Never mind that these young athletes are beating marks the Robert
Spetzlers set a quarter century ago. The point is, *they are beating his marks.*

Spetzler points to Curtis Dickman, concluding as chief resident, as an
example of the new neurosurgeon. His vita lists forty-eight publications,
twenty-nine in refereed journals; of the twenty-nine, he is lead author
on twenty-one. He has written five textbook chapters, two as lead author,
three as second to Sonntag. He has been hired as the neurosurgical partnership's tenth member, making it one of the larger such groups in the
country. Dickman will be charged with establishing a research program on
spinal cord injuries, complementing Zabramski's in vascular neurosurgery.

Spetzler still gets the lion's share of what Wilson called "the marbles."
St. Joseph's Hospital and Medical Center is about to undertake an expansion estimated to cost in the $200 million range, which will include increased
laboratory space and many more beds, and this in a period when hospitals
are generally retrenching. Neurosurgery now commands five operating
rooms—more, Spetzler says, than anywhere else in the country—and after
the expansion it will have six. But he would not want still-more OR space
because he believes the unity of Barrow as a single entity would diminish.

He is concerned that BNI not grow too large, fearing it would lose
the quality it has achieved by bringing together top neurosurgeons
in subspecialties as they are needed.

FROM HERE THE FUTURE seems increasingly determinate for Spetzler,
and if that is usually intolerable to the restless spirit, he gives no signs of being
disturbed by it. Neurosurgery would proceed by its small advances, he said,
new techniques and new tools making rescues possible that now are only
thinkable, then making them commonplace; virtuoso approaches and procedures would be enhanced by new technologies so they spread throughout
the world of neurosurgery. The major area of advance for the remainder of
the decade, hence of the century and millennium, would be in robotics.
Devices like the wand would enable all neurosurgeons to foresee where they
are proceeding literally, rather than metaphorically by their own "inner vision."
Similarly, robotics would allow ever more precise control in placing clips or

tissue, the operator's hands and eyes increasingly extended by tech-nology. But the neurosurgeon still towers at the center of all this, because judgment remains the critical determinant of success. The power of decision remains in these hands, which move with ever-increasing finesse until—Surprise.

Looking down the road, Spetzler sees a shocking discontinuity, a break in the steady incremental progress of his medical specialty. He sees the end of neurosurgery. Not in his professional career, but in his lifetime. Scientists see order in the muddle of chaos, referring to the rise of new regularities as emergent properties; conversely they see discontinuities in the middle of order, sudden yawning chasms that are, ironically, born of that order. It is just such a discontinuity Spetzler sees in neurosurgery's not-distant future. Not in the year 2000, but perhaps twenty years into that new century, a vision of 2020.

"I see the spectacular procedures of today giving way to treatments for diseases like Parkinson's or Alzheimer's disease," Spetzler says. "The neuro-surgeon will implant cultured cells that will restore the function of destroyed tissue. Today we are acting against lesions and illnesses *threatening* healthy tissue. But once tissue is destroyed and function is lost, there is nothing we can do. That's what I see coming—the restoration of lost function. And I'm not talking about fetal cell implantation," he says, referring to the controversial attempts to implant brain tissue of aborted fetuses to restore Parkinson's patients.

"Fetal cells are just a bridge. It should not be long before cultured cell lines can be implanted to restore brain function." The advances in genetic engineering should make it possible for neuroscientists to clone healthy brain tissue, grow it in laboratory cultures, and pass it along to neurosurgeons for implantation, the result being recovery of destroyed brain function. "That will be the neurosurgeon's job—restoring lost abilities," he says.

The effects of such new powers will make neurosurgeons ever more successful in the short term, but in the long term such advances will eliminate their defining role—life and death judgment.

"If you can grow the portion of the brain that's diseased, and if you have robotics that are exquisite in placing the tissue, then the decision-making tree that the neurosurgeon is intimately involved with today becomes less a part of his or her existence. In that case, the true predictor of success will be the ability to grow the right cell lines to put out the appropriate factors, and the placement will be less critical."

Eventually Spetzler sees the field at a critical juncture in which the neuro-surgeon "is more like a mechanic, using robotics and other technological advances to place healthy tissue precisely where it is needed."

Like a mechanic? This from the classical pianist, the breaker of horses, the virtuoso who offered condolences to the search committee that failed to pick him as a chairman? Yes.

"Neurosurgeons will play a critical role in bringing all this about," Spetzler says, and in doing so may put themselves out of business. But, "It is not an unglorious occupation to put yourself out of business. That requires all of the very best talents. The sin is to try to hang onto the past only to have a profession, rather than using discoveries to make a glorious step into the future, to be part of whatever comes next."

Spetzler points out that history is full of lost arts. "We don't have a lot of blacksmiths anymore, and every village had one. We really don't have general practitioners anymore, no matter how hard we keep trying to bring them back."

To be sure, the neurosurgical "type" will not go out of existence, because it is a personality driven to be part of "whatever comes next." Nor does Spetzler believe his current crop of residents will find themselves reduced to technicians—but he does think that such talented individuals may find themselves working under different titles.

"Think about the qualities we consider necessary for a good neuro-surgeon," he says. "A certain temperament, a certain decisiveness. A certain ego skill that allows you to compensate for dramatic failures as well as dramatic successes. Society right now sees the neurosurgeon as a physician having those qualities.

"But what's next? As we emerge into this new era, such an individual may be the head of a clinical laboratory that makes the decisions about who gets what treatment, and who oversees the creation and growth of the tissues and factors needed. So maybe this personality type, who now becomes a neuro-surgeon, then will become the head of such a clinical or basic science laboratory."

SO SAID SPETZLER IN 1992. But reality continued contra-dicting him in the most complimentary ways, putting his predictions in bold relief. A future that did not clamor for the best neurosurgeons was plainly not at hand, and his own international reputation was growing daily. One standstill prompted a long, lavishly illustrated feature focusing on Spetzler and his family in the leading French magazine *Figaro*.

Consider "outcome": If the patient comes in a rocket scientist, does he go home a rocket scientist? The question would be tested on a writer. Not just any writer, but a world-famous writer whose newspaper column embodied his self-created persona as New York incarnate. If he comes in with a brain that is witty, irascible, tough, then in a flash poignant, senti-mental, sad, and, in another flash, howlingly funny, will he emerge that way? And will the pieces fit together right? That's a lot of subtle magic to send away and then call back again.

Jimmy Breslin was the name: writer of *The Gang That Couldn't Shoot Straight* and ten other books, Pulitzer-Prize winning columnist, and a humorous protest candidate with Norman Mailer for vice mayor and mayor of the Big Apple. Breslin did not have a standstill at Barrow, but he was taken down into a deep barbiturate coma so that Spetzler could repair an aneurysm of the anterior communicating artery—"A-com." Ironically, the aneurysm was asypmtomatic. Breslin had an MRI because his left eyelid drooped as a side effect of diabetes. That illness had caused palsy of the oculomotor nerve, which controls movement of the eyes. The MRI disclosed the large aneurysm nearly touching the optic nerve.

If Breslin did not come back all the way, his losses would be obvious to more than family and friends. Several million readers would know it or would never see his work again. Searching New York for the best surgeon in the world to handle his problem, Breslin hit Spetzler's name at every turn.

Above all, Breslin worried about what not coming back all the way would mean to him. Would he be able to recognize a joke? Would he feel? And for him, of singular importance, would he be the writer he had been from his teenage years until a week earlier? He did not want to die—and he believed God had decided it was not his time. But he wondered if dying might not be better than losing his gift with words.

The personality, the person, is not an entity that sits in one place in the brain, where it can be protected. Self represents the highest integrated set of functions in the brain. So said George Prigatano, Barrow's Director of Neuropsychology. It was he who observed Jack Schulte's inability to initiate action. It is he who examines those emerging from neurotrauma and neuro-surgery, judging to what extent they truly become themselves again.

You can pass every test of the Glasgow Coma Scale and not be yourself again. How do you know if you are? Most often you, the patient, do not. Family members notice. The patient believes he or she can do everything the same as before, sometimes with disastrous results. Those close can tell what is missing.

Who you are is not a neat set of brain functions, nor a finite combination of emanations of brain structures. Yet all of those plainly feed into the creation of the self, and the loss of them means loss of self, or awareness of self. The person, soul, mind seems to represent what neuroscientists call emergent properties of brain activity—properties that truly do not exist in microcosm at the cellular level, and which emerge only at higher levels. That is the end of resolution, down where the brain is multi-billions of cells, each cell comprising parts, linking with incoming and outgoing chemical messengers, receiving and sending chemical messages.

The concept of an emergent self runs counter to the idea of resolution; it is a whole that cannot be summed from its parts. Look at the dazzling sun called mind; try to increase the resolution, and it vanishes. The mind, for all we might talk of its "parts," is indivisible, a wonder of aspects and perspectives without limit, yet irreducible to any of the cellular roots that give it life.

But damage parts of the deep cortical structures of the limbic system and the emotions that give weight and meaning to the world are not the same. Lose the tip of one temporal lobe containing the structure called the hippocampus and nothing permanent happens. However, if both temporal lobe tips are destroyed in an accident, a person emerges who cannot lay down new memories. The sufferer lives in a permanent present tense incapable of foreseeing anything or of remembering anything that occurred after the injury, yet with all memories before injury perfectly intact.

A few weeks after surgery, Breslin began halting, frustrating efforts to write again. His coming back all the way was both proved and hailed in his memoir, *I Want To Thank My Brain For Remembering Me*. In the book, published by Little, Brown in 1996, Breslin reports on his surgery, through interviews with Spetzler and his crew, and recalls articulately, humorously, movingly, the life that had come before and would follow. Same old Breslin.

Such cases put the spotlight on Spetzler. But he has always made it clear that it is BNI's institutional reputation that concerns him most, and there was evidence that was growing as well. As Jimmy Breslin began his slow recovery, a whole floor of BNI was being converted, literally, into a hotel for visiting royalty. The Queen Mother of Saudi Arabia had come with an entourage of dozens of family members and staff for spinal surgery by Volker Sonntag.

Spetzler always said he had no desire to leave Barrow, ever. Where it goes, he would go.

Others who know him were never so positive.

"It's not a question of whether Barrow is the top," said a fellow chairman. "It's a question of whether, some day, Robert Spetzler thinks there is some place he can make higher. In that case I wouldn't presume to bet on what he would do."

Reality equals outcome. But when *is* the outcome, finally?

CHERYL DURAN HAD MET MICHAEL JONES on a blind date in May 1992. She was a divorced mother of two young boys, still on good terms with their father, with whom she shared custody. Michael was a construction worker who had been driving through Arizona on a cross-country tour with a Marine reserve buddy two years earlier, visited an uncle, and decided he liked the place. The place was Wickenburg, in the mountainous desert northwest of Phoenix, a town world famous for its dude ranches. They married in October 1993 in the Community Alliance Church, where both were active and devoted members. Past tense. The past all seems compressed to her now, kneaded and foreshortened so that everything is recent.

The new year 1995 opened bursting with promise. Cheryl was pregnant with their first child, and Michael had completed construction plans for the home they would build with their own hands, not far from the small rental they had occupied since they their marriage. All they needed were the stamps of the building inspector and approval of a loan. Cheryl had a good job as a mental-health technician at an eating-disorder treatment center; Michael had steady work as a drywall installer in the booming town.

At 5 a.m., February 7, getting ready for work, Cheryl was slammed with a monster headache. Then she threw up. She couldn't walk for the pain splitting her head. All of it came without a warning, like something out of a bad-pregnancy story, and this had been a tough pregnancy from the start. Was it a legendary bout of morning sickness? Her speech was slurred and confused. Michael called her mother, Sarene, who lived nearby. Sarene didn't think the violent attack could be caused solely by pregnancy. Cheryl herself had just finished a CPR course, and now she seemed to have every bad symptom she had learned about. Michael called their obstetrician and had him paged, but decided not to wait for the call-back. He bundled Cheryl into their car, and they left for the local hospital.

Twelve hours later, all she could remember was spending the whole day in tears. Everything was lost. Dr. Robert Spetzler was telling her that she needed brain surgery for an aneurysm. And Spetzler was telling Michael she would need a standstill procedure, a cardiac arrest. He explained what that meant, paused to let it settle in. Then he went on. They would not only stop her heart but drain her blood. The risk would be high, but there was no less-risky alternative. The pregnancy was another matter; Spetzler did not believe the fetus could survive and wanted them to understand.

Michael interrupted for the only time, asking Spetzler only to be concerned with taking care of his wife and leaving God to take care of the baby.

Research had to be done quickly. Babies had been taken from the womb after their mothers' deaths, but they were full-term, ready to be born. As of 1995, no fetus had undergone such a procedure at all, so there was no precedent.

Dr. Stephan Cardon, who had just joined BNI as a neuroanesthesiologist, needed to do research on his own. The majority of anesthesia drugs were all right for pregnant women; he needed to eliminate those that were not. As the procedure began, Cardon's colleagues were pessimistic. The cardiac perfusionist, who would be responsible for circulating and cooling Jones's blood, as well as for shutting off and restarting the pumps, foresaw certain miscarriage.

At the last moment, Cardon was able to hook up an ultrasound machine to Jones. As a result, this standstill moved along with two images on the 3-D monitor: the view through the intraoperative microscope, and, inset, the visualized beating of a ten-week-old heart. Then the bypass pumps were turned on, her heart was stopped, and chilled blood began circulating through her. The blurry beating went on. And the chilling deepened, and the pumps went off. Now, as always in standstill, the patient monitors fell silent and went flatline. The ultrasound went on, swelling and dropping, never missing a beat and slowing only slightly. When Spetzler said, "Pumps on," after twenty minutes, the relief in the room was audible. But what was the outcome?

Spetzler told Michael Jones that the odds of the baby's being normal were very difficult to judge. Abortion was an option, he said. Although it could not be done at St. Joseph's, a Catholic hospital, he could refer the couple. But abortion was not an option for them, Michael said. So the difficult decisions were over. TV cameras rolled again. Here was a beautiful mother, a heart-beating sonogram, a miracle rescue of a young woman, another first for a standstill.

But what was the outcome? Off-camera, Cheryl Jones plunged into torment that grew worse with passing months. Used to taking care of her home and two children, now she was virtually immobilized. Stunned by the aid that poured in from friends, church members, strangers, she was simultaneously overwhelmed by feelings of gratitude and uselessness. She could barely walk, and then only wearing a cumbersome brace to support her right leg. Her entire right side was partially paralyzed.

Depression set in, far beyond the level that sometimes overcomes expectant mothers, even those enduring difficult pregnancies. Why? There is a lot of mystery in how the combination of anesthesia, lack of oxygen and the hormonal changes of pregnancy can combine to undo what the mind has so carefully built. Cheryl became suicidal. She despaired for the baby's well-being, she felt her sanity slipping, she saw no hope.

The ending is simple enough to tell but there's still plenty of mystery in the how and why. Cheryl's obstetrician, Dr. Edward Sattenspiel, found a combination of anti-depressants that evened her out. She didn't even *feel better*, she recalled; she just didn't feel so hopeless. Yet those aren't both feelings in the same sense of the word. And anyway, how did a certain combination of chemicals reverse a complex mental tailspin? Why do they sometimes fail? No answers, not at the level we like answers. Such explanations as there are involve changes in the actions of complex molecules called neurotransmitters—brain messengers. But the changes in outcome represented by minor alterations in micro-molecules are life-altering.

Three weeks before the baby was due, Cheryl's water broke. The Joneses found themselves on another hair-raising dash from Wickenburg to Phoenix, skittering into St. Joseph's parking lot just after midnight, August 18. Adam Michael Jones was born at 6:06 a.m. He seemed perfectly okay. Cheryl was home the next day and beginning to take care of the baby, two children and house. And here would be a great place to ring down the curtain on this story, if there were such a gift for calling endings.

Three weeks into fatherhood, Michael Jones was working on a construction job at a golf resort in Wickenburg. He had put a six-foot stepladder atop a six-foot scaffold and climbed to the top of the assembly carrying drywall. Suddenly the whole thing collapsed, pitching him into the ground. Now he was the one rushed by ambulance to St. Joseph's.

A few days later Michael was wheeled into BNI surgery, as Volker Sonntag's patient. He had severely fractured two vertebrae in his lower back and possibly damaged his spinal cord, how badly still unknown. It was a far more complex procedure than most back surgeries. Sonntag had to approach the spinal column through the left side of Michael's chest in order to fuse bones where the thoracic spine, from which the ribs emanate, becomes the lumbar spine of the lower back. Michael might not walk, or he might have suffered brain damage from swelling and not recover from that. Cheryl sat quietly in the neurosurgery waiting room, her family and Michael's gathered around her, a basket decorated in blue bunting at her feet. Its occupant slept quietly. Today was September 15 and, to quote a dark joke, just as the light had shone at the end of the tunnel, a train appeared behind it. The most neutral observer would have to say that, for the Joneses, 1995 had been one hell of a year. But Cheryl Jones was remarkably composed, direct, determined. Come what may, she was herself again.

OUT OF SURGERY and into the blaze July. Phoenix is burning, rising in waves like a light tapestry in the hot wind. Consider reality, that magnificent artifice of the brain. See how the desert world wavers without definition or contrast, its darknesses heated to light earth tones, its whiteness beyond color. The visual world is ambiguous, coming in shaky, uncertain waves. The sky is without color. Light reflects off heat waves as though off water, and the world thus seen in reflection is only a little less clear than a straight-on look at daylight. Reality meltdown. But the brain puts all these shaky clues together and pronounces the world okay; damned uncomfortable but nothing for concern. So Phoenix rises on a sultry afternoon; so do visions of cathedrals and neurological institutes. So do mirages.

The doctor says these cases were cured. Were they? Doctor A says this patient is gone. Is she? Robert Spetzler says this fascinating amalgam of spirit and stone, physical plant and concept, called Barrow Neurological Institute, is the best in the world. Is it? Reality is not simple; that is not new. The ways reality has gotten complicated are strange; sometimes it seems there are only mirages holding steadier or less so for varying amounts of time. And if that's so, we know whom to blame—the brain, creator of the mind that is its own place. Or maybe it's the other way around.

So ENDED *THE HEALING BLADE* the first time around. But stories don't end with story-tellers' deadlines. They roll on behind the curtain, if you dare to look again. Fast forward and Phoenix still rises apparition-like in the heat of another July, much the same and much different. A $40-million research building appears where the BNI parking lot used to be. It concentrates all of the institute's research efforts in one place and expands them manyfold. Research in neurology has expanded, but the focus is still, always, on neurosurgery. The building houses a gamma knife, the latest gleaming, high-tech weapon against lesions deep in the brain. Perhaps the gamma knife is a harbinger of Spetzler's forecast. Operated by a neurosurgeon, it burns out tumors and may be useful for arteriovenous malformations—AVMs— non-invasively, without an entry wound of any kind. This $6 million machine is one of a handful in the country, and the only one south of Denver and west of Houston. More of that later.

Today, drive from St. Joseph's downtown to Interstate 10 and head west.

Beyond where the last suburbs vanish in the whited-out desert, turn north through the Vulture Mountains, and soon you reach Wickenburg.

JULY 18, 1997

Cheryl and Michael Jones still rent the small house on Bowman Barn, a dirt road whose cul de sac they share with the parking lot of a plumbing supply store. The fenced-off house with its lawn and trees and its greenery dotted with toys is its own enclave, and they are a cheerful clan. As soon as the visitor is seated, Adam Michael dances rapidly up and down, pumping his legs with the enthusiasm of an almost-two-year-old with a bright idea. He rushes from the room and back in an instant, holding his book of children's Bible stories.

"Read!" he says.

"In a few minutes, okay?"

"Read!"

"When we're done talking," Cheryl says firmly.

"Read!" undeterrable.

So we begin, "In the beginning...." And within a minute he's had enough of that and darts off to play.

"He's *really* two already," Cheryl sighs. "He even says 'no' when you ask him about something he wants."

Cheryl's two older boys, now twelve and nine, are out for the afternoon.

"I'm a much better person for all of this. We both are," she says of their long ordeal. "When the surgery was over, I think I was in denial about what had almost happened. Then it hit me that I had nearly died—in a way, did die—and I realized everything that could still go wrong. I got terribly depressed. The surgery was the hard time for the family. Recovering was the terrible time for me."

The new-house plans were approved by the city and their loan came through within days of each other—unfortunately, two weeks after Michael broke his back. He spent fourteen months out of work. "We've had to put those on hold," Michael says, but they are still ready to go whenever their finances permit, and their lot a mile away is waiting. They are less surprised by the amount of their debt than by the generosity of those they owe.

"People we knew and people we never heard of wrote to me and sent us gifts and money," Cheryl says. "It was amazing. I'll never forget it."

They fell thousands of dollars behind in their rent, Michael says, and their landlord let them slide until he was able to return to work more than a year later. They owed the grocer and "everyone else in town," but no one complained.

Both are now "sort of recovered." Cheryl still feels some weakness in her right hand, not noticeable to others and noticeable even to her only at times, and the hand is growing steadily stronger. Michael still has back pain that limits how strenuously he can work.

The couple came through trials that would sink many families. They say their faith is stronger; and their survivors' sense of humor plainly is.

Michael says, "We used to joke about whose surgery cost more."

"Mine did," Cheryl concludes.

"But I have more metal inside," he says.

One evening during an especially rugged period last year, Michael sat contemplating "what direction the Lord was planning for my life," when suddenly a dazzling burst of light appeared at the window. He thought it might be an omen, but their cat, "Spetzy," had touched a live wire and nearly been electrocuted. After expensive trips to the vet, the cat suddenly vanished into the desert, probably fallen prey to a coyote. "I decided not to be looking so much for signs," he says laughing. In another month he plans to go into construction on his own.

As bad as things were, Michael says, a far worse outcome for Cheryl probably was avoided. "Dr. Spetzler thinks the aneurysm may have developed when she had her first children," he says. "If it had gone then, or later when she was in labor with Adam, it probably would have killed her on the spot."

Finally, a few months ago, Cheryl began getting severe headaches. Worried, the couple headed into Phoenix again for a series of scans. This time the scans came up clear. Sometimes a headache is only a headache, and the outcome is unchanged.

t e n # Emergence

THE MEDICAL AUDIENCE IS SEATED,
the slide-projector fan hums the prelude. "Lights, please," Spetzler says.
The introductory message announces:

CLINICAL MANAGEMENT OF GIANT CRANIAL ANEURYSMS

BARROW NEUROLOGICAL INSTITUTE

"May I have the next slide please."

A glistening opalescent balloon, a familiar image by now, swells out of
the dark. Sometimes by becoming familiar, the unknown loses its terrors.
Not this time. The great pinkish-gray blob becomes more fearful with each
articulation, the devastation it can cause becoming clearer with each example.

"The hallmark of an aneurysm that has become symptomatic is that
unforgettable headache," Spetzler says. "The sentinel headache, the one that's
different than any other headache they've ever had, is very important."

Slides of aneurysms glide past, blossoming. Then, clipped with their tiny,
fancy clothespins they lie stripped of danger, harmless. By the date of one
slide, that might be Jennifer Turner's aneurysm going by. But then comes
a view of another brain, this one ruined and dark, the mind's rich farmland

under the black lava of a burst aneurysm—"an absolutely devastating condition," Spetzler says.

Sometimes the patient survives and looks good, and the surgeon "will sort of pat himself or herself on the back and say, 'What a great result,' because the patient moves everything and the neurological exam is normal. The family will come back in three months and say, 'Where is my husband or my wife that I've been married to?'" Gone. How can so much remain yet all that's humanly important vanish like vapor?

If an aneurysm ruptures during surgery, as it is released from the compress of surrounding brain, the expert neurosurgeon often can bring bleeding under control. But the odds are not good, the surgeon "trying to look down with high magnification... in eloquent territory, and you've got blood spurting up at you, blocking your vision. Disaster is almost assured."

Now here is one major point of this talk, a rescue: the standstill. We see an operating field clear and without pressure and note the contrast with that angry, inflamed bulb. There is Jim Youngblood's aneurysm on the February day he turned forty-eight, his rebirth-day. "Next slide." Cheryl Jones, ten weeks pregnant with hardly a hope for her fetus, if even for herself. Now mother and child.

"...the patient can survive without any circulation, without any blood pressure—therefore no bleeding if you open the aneurysm—for up to an hour."

At BNI, "We have by far the largest experience in the world of modern hypothermic cardiac standstill. We have sixty-four patients that we've treated" during standstill.

THE WORLD OF 1997 is smaller by far than that of 1992. Spetzler gave this talk in June at an international congress in Amsterdam, the Netherlands. Afterward a surgeon approached as a potential patient. A few weeks later Spetzler responded to his first E-mail referral, from Nepal. The surgeon had the largest skull-base aneurysm Spetzler had ever seen. Standstill was scheduled forAugust. On July 23 Spetzler gave virtually the same talk in Yuma, Arizona, in part to alert diagnosticians to watch for "that sentinel headache." But in part he flew to Yuma to protect BNI's medical territory. The rules of medicine have been changed by managed care and the increased competition for specialty dollars.

A major neurological institute must reach to Nepal and take care of Yuma, but even then it will never find the security that once seemed a given. It's an uncertain new world at sixty-four standstills and counting.

WEDNESDAY, JULY 23, 1997
   MORNING: 7:30 EASTERN DAYLIGHT TIME.
             4:30 MOUNTAIN STANDARD TIME.

DEBRA AND DANIEL LAWSON, mother and son, leave home in Knoxville, Tennessee to board their flight, bound for Phoenix but unfortunately requiring a plane change in Atlanta. Severe morning thunderstorms over Georgia rock the plane and leave Debra feeling her head will split open. But this is no sentinel headache, like none she's ever had before. Blond, thirty-eight years old, fashion-plate slim, Debra Lawson has suffered from crippling migraines most of her life. There is more than a hint of the familial flaw here, though the connection is not clear. Her family tree has several migraine sufferers and at least two deaths by brain hemorrhage. For years Lawson has been on state disability, a waitress laid low by the headaches. Tennessee provided the scans that revealed to Spetzler "as bad an aneurysm in eloquent territory as you have ever seen, as dangerous as they come."

Eloquent territory. A terrifically descriptive expression in the trade jargon of the neurosurgeon. In discourse, eloquence refers to the powerfully expressive, speech that is not only vivid but moves its listeners. The eloquent is both articulate and powerful. Down in the skull base, along the bone-platform behind the eyes called the fossa that serves as the major support for the flat bottom of the brain, behind and above the circle of Willis, lies the brain's most protected territory. And its most eloquent. Expressive of all the commands that keep us conscious as well as thinking and feeling; powerful as the life signals that emanate, flowing to the rest of the brain, the heart, the lungs.

On Friday, Debra Lawson will become BNI standstill number sixty-five. Today she will head for a terrific family reunion. Her mother died when she was five years old, and she has hardly known her sisters because of age differences and the frequent moves so common in recent decades. Today she will stay at the home of Ray and Joann Smith. Joann is a sister she has only rarely seen since childhood.

At 4:30 a.m., Cody Lossing begins his rounds of the six Barrow operating rooms, all eerily quiet and squeaky clean. For the first three hours of his shift Monday through Thursday, the scrub tech's job is to make sure that they are indeed squeaky clean, as they should have been left the day before, and stocked with the many parcels that equip each room. Each room must be set up with instrument trays for craniotomy, that is, opening of the cranial vault; laminectomy, opening the bony spinal canal, and soft-tissue surgery, involving brain tissue itself. Each room's case cart must contain cottonoids, razors, shampoo and tape for prep; and Major A and B packs, which contain disposable scalpels, towels and suctioning devices. He must make sure there is still film and videotape loaded in the intraoperative filming devices. The circulating nurse on the first case will check out the scope itself.

The sinks between each pair of ORs are the responsibility of the hospital cleaning staffers. They will place scrubbing soap in the dispenses and stock the shelves with three different kinds of face mask. Everyone stepping into the OR must have a mask, but visitors just dropping in with a message, or checking on an opening, or carrying away a tumor sample, can grab one of the stiff fiber masks held in place by an elastic band—easy on, easy off, but not comfortable if you are spending all day inside. Those manning the desk in the hallway or the sterilizing room or Pam Smith's photo office don't need masks. They emerge from the men's and women's dressing rooms in the minimum attire permitted in the operating suite: blue scrubs, a choice of one of three kinds of caps, and fiber "clean" booties that mask the sound of footfalls even on the busiest day.

Working the ORs this shift is like working outside before dawn. First there is silence so total it's palpable. And at some point you seem never to notice, day sounds come up singly, then in pairs, then patterns, and suddenly it's 7:00 a.m. and clamor is everywhere. Terry Steinberg, the operating room manager, is going over schedules with Barbara McWilliams and Tina Lucero, who manage the front desk, take calls, page, answer questions, match cases with the schedule. The board opposite their desk begins filling up the afternoon before, and by early morning is often a patchwork of erasure and chalking-over.

In the sterilizing room, Frances Rocha has gotten the first tests done on her sterilization equipment, making sure that the oven-like washers themselves have passed their "Biological Attest"—that they are free of microbes.

From early in the morning until mid-afternoon, she will scramble to stay even with the ORs. On a typical day, she and her assistants will run fifteen to eighteen loads of instruments, most of them highest grade stainless steel, through ultrasound and steam, and that can add up to as many as three thousand pieces.

At day's end, by 7:30 p.m., she and her crew will make sure the bipolar cauteries, remote control wires and any instruments containing electric cords or plastic that can't take the boiling heat are shipped downstairs. There, another crew will put them through an eight-hour sterilizing bath of ethylene oxide followed by four hours of air drying. In the morning Rocha will make sure all those sets have joined her sterilized stainless-steel instruments marked for their proper rooms. She is also ready to "flash" instruments that may have been dropped—to put them through intense, pressurized steam to sterilize them quickly.

Each day is similar. First silence, then clatter, finally a din, cacophony that must be resolved into its symphonies. And rounds. The occasional canon. And rarely a fugue. The rooms will run all day and, these days, well into the night. It is usually 11:30 p.m. before the last elective surgery is done, the patient wheeled into recovery, the OR scrubbed, disinfected, and covered for tomorrow, the instruments shipped away for cleaning, the silence total again.

Noon

IN OR 2, CURTIS DICKMAN, last seen passing from senior resident to attending neurosurgeon as a member of the Barrow partnership, is operating on a difficult back problem, a degenerating disk that requires a two-stage surgery. The procedure involves decompressing the spinal cord, which is being pinched because of the disk's deterioration, and attaching two vertebral bones together with plates and screws, to keep proper separation between them, which the disk had originally provided. Once considered the routine end of neurosurgery, the spinal subspecialty has become exciting.

There are new devices and techniques, new ways to restore peripheral nerve function. Competition also has intensified, because back surgery is among the few neurological operations often done by orthopedic surgeons—bone specialists—and therefore neurosurgeons are put in direct competition with them, in an already tough climate.

Spinal surgery is also the subject of excitement because research is approaching ways to make real its ages-old dream of regenerating a severed spinal cord and restoring movement to paralyzed limbs. Spetzler thinks that could take thirty years or more, but if it is done, even quadriplegics might walk again. For now, some of the most dramatic advances in neurosurgery were pioneered in spinal operations. Endoscopes, thin fiber-optic tubes that carry light in and microscope images out, permit many procedures to be carried out with tiny incisions instead of massive entry wounds. Endoscopic surgery, such as Dickman performs today, has decreased recovery time so dramatically that patients often go home the day after complex operations. There is talk in the near future of same-day departures in neurosurgery, where hospital recoveries now are commonly measured in weeks.

Such changes, of course, have major economic importance, but there is far greater benefit. Tiny incisions radically reduce the danger of infection, which is still the number one cause of morbidity in post-operative patients. Dickman has been doing endoscopic spinal surgery since joining the staff.

But the star performer in OR 2 this afternoon is not Dickman but his new assistant. Dickman's eyes are pressed to the intraoperative microscope, his hands poised with dissector over the open incision that exposes the bony vertebrae he is working on.

"Move up," Dickman says, and strong arms move the scope up for him. "Move down," and the scope moves down a bit, seen in 3D in the color monitor. The 3D glasses, once the exciting new teaching tools of the OR, now are routine, and so improved that the image on-screen seems more reality than video. Now Dickman says briskly, "Set position 1."

"Position 1 set," comes the reply in the soft female voice familiar to air travelers, elevator riders, and some car owners. It is the voice of the computer, this version named AESOP, silky yet firm, in perfect control.

"AESOP move up." Up she goes. Or rather, it goes. Disconcerting. "Stop."

It halts.

"Set Position 2."

"Position 2 set." The computer in this session now recognizes two positions by name, as well as a whole series of commands, and it can make finer movements of the endoscope's controls than all but the most dexterous human. Dickman points out that AESOP isn't doing any part of the surgery; it is just providing him another set of hands. Among those looking on are two company representatives who hope to sell the device to St. Joseph's for $50,000. Dickman wears a headset microphone, the only hint that he is not speaking to a human.

"Go to Position 1." AESOP's arms move the scope precisely to Position 1. "Move up.... Move left... Stop. Go to Position 2."

"Position 2," says the voice, the scope moving back to pre-arranged Position 2.

AESOP is hardly cutting edge these days. Its robotics technology has been around for years. Similarly, software has been on the market for several years that allows computers to take dictation by learning a user's voice. To use AESOP, each neurosurgeon carries a wallet-sized computer card virtually indistinguishable from those popped into a laptop slot for telecommunications. That computer card contains his or her voice print. But AESOP— Automatic Endoscopic System for Optimal Positioning—is the tip of the iceberg.

Company rep Sam Danna explains, "By next year we expect to be marketing our Zeus system, and the Zeus robots actually operate."

That is a leap in more than technology; it raises issues of responsibility and control, ethical questions that are not easily answered. But like all such difficult questions, these arise out of a shining promise. The Zeus robots can be geared down to microscopic standards. A surgeon whose hands are half as good as those of a Spetzler or Ojemann or Heros potentially can be just as steady, just as fine, just as able to endure long hours with a bipolar cautery suspended over eloquent real estate, then threading a shadow with a cobweb. The surgeon's hand moves a centimeter; Zeus translates it to a millimeter. The future Spetzler had predicted seemed far off if not farfetched; five years later it is here.

But not quite. Spetzler's daily operating load is enormous, and they are all cases only he or a few of the world's best can do. Scores of his cases, like the one across the hall in OR 1 this afternoon, come with medical jackets full of opinions that conclude simply: inoperable. And then he operates.

The new tools of neurosurgery show themselves best in these "inoperable" cases.

By 12:30 in the afternoon, Spetzler is in the middle of a tumor of staggering proportions. On the MRI scan it looks like a wad of cotton, bounded but indistinct, pure white, obliterating the middle of the brain and jamming shut the ventricles. The navigational wand introduced five years ago is now used daily. As Spetzler and Chief Resident Dean Karahalios operate, one or the other frequently places the wand on a landmark on the patient's skull. On an adjacent monitor they can see a three-dimensional display of the composite scans showing precisely where they are, and how close to the tumor border they have reached with their probing with cautery and dissector.

Spetzler is scheduled to fly out in two and a half hours to speak to the medical staff of Yuma Regional Medical Center, but for all that intrudes on the concentration in the OR, the trip might as well be days away. A specimen of tumor is sent down to neuropathology, and the team continues working.

From a visitor's point of view, the most remarkable addition to neurosurgery is the third dimension added by the holographic-seeming displays. That third dimension was dramatic enough seen in the surface furrows of the brain lobes. Now, wearing the latest version of glasses, as the neurosurgeons move deeper and deeper into the brain to remove tumor, the depth is breathtaking and the detail and color perfect. Watching the giant monitor, there is a striking sense of "virtual reality," that you are climbing down into the recesses of the brain, blue and red cables everywhere and, forcing its way through, the irregular tumor mass, blurry and without definition in this exquisitely defined world.

The phone rings. Stephen Coons in neuropathology has identified the tumor as a meningioma. That is, it originated in and of the meninges that cover and protect the brain. All brain tumors are dangerous, but this is among the least so because it is not invasive; if not removed, its growing pressure will kill the patient, but the tumor will not infiltrate and destroy other brain tissue. Surgery can be a cure.

At 1:10 the phone rings again. Spetzler's secretary, Paula Ohlwiler, reminds him through the nurse who answers that he is booked on the 2:10 flight to Yuma. But this neurosurgery, delayed by an emergency this morning, has bumped the flight. "See if there's another way to get there later. A private flight if nothing else."

The anesthesia monitor is beeping irregularly, not in the steady tattoo of a pulse. "Why is the cranial nerve monitor going off?" Spetzler asks, a question to the residents.

"Nerves 3 and 5 are being irritated," says one. Cranial Nerve 3 is the oculomotor nerve. Signals from the brain running along its cables activate the muscles that move the eyes. Cranial Nerve 5 is the trigeminal. Syndromes involving severe facial pain result from its inflammation.

"Why are we getting signals from there?"

And the residents respond, slowly. They point out CN 3 and CN 5, large and glossy cables running through these deepening interiors. The cranial nerves are close to the probing instruments, and the electronic alerts to the anesthesiologist signal what would be pain messages if the patient were awake. Hard as they are trying to avoid it, their work to free tissues from the tumor is irritating these cranial nerves.

It is now 1:40. So much for the 2:10 to Yuma. Another call comes in: How about the 3:10 flight? "Possibly," he says. In fact by 2:30 the tumor is excised and closing has begun. Spetzler scrubs out of the OR, moments later is dressing in his inner office, in another moment emerges suited— but tieless. "See if one of the residents or someone has a spare tie," he says. Ohlwiler hunts up a dark-red striped tie, and he is off to the airport.

What are the chances for the meningioma patient? "I fully expect a complete recovery and a normal life," he says. "I believe we got it all, and this [tumor type] is very slow growing in any case. It's hard to believe she was asymptomatic, but she was, so there's no reason to think there will be deficits" in her brain function or abilities or personality. There is reason, in other words, to see a cure where four hours earlier a giant tumor all but obliterated the center of a young woman's brain.

And we are off to Yuma and serious business of a different kind, soon bouncing hard through the daily afternoon thermal currents of a rainless summer, following the ribbon of Interstate 8 toward the Colorado River and Yuma.

These are terrifically successful days for Spetzler. Three years ago, at age 49, he was named "Honored Guest" by the Congress of Neurological Surgeons at its annual meeting. Like the peaks of achievement in many professions, this one goes by an unassuming name. But it is an honor to which the best neurosurgeons aspire and few attain. In the previous ten years before Spetzler's name was added, the names included Walter Dandy (posthumously), Cushing's protégé and rival; Gazi Yasargil of Zurich, the pioneer of microneurosurgery and Spetzler's mentor; Thor Sundt, of the Mayo Clinic, who soon after the honor would lose his valiant fight with cancer; Charles Wilson of UCSF; Bennett Stein of Columbia; Robert Ojemann of MGH. They are all the senior members of the world elite in neurosurgery, at or near retirement; Spetzler was the first of the next generation to be honored. He was the only person under 50 ever named, among awardees whose average age was 63.

The Barrow partnership has been expanded to include top former residents—not only Dickman but Kris Smith, earlier pointed out as perhaps the most promising neurosurgical resident ever at Barrow; and as BNI pushed into Scottsdale and the turf of the Mayo Clinic there, it added Brian Fitzpatrick and Frederick Marciano.

But one could easily look forward from 1992 and see a straight path to 1997. That would be a false trajectory. Spetzler's being here at Barrow would have happily shocked many of the staff just a year ago. And a year before that as well. The same neurological institutes that Spetzler had talked about over the years before had come wooing him and Sonntag as a team in the same relationship they enjoyed here.

First, Stanford made an offer for them to become director and vice director of neurosurgery. BNI kept him by bettering the offer and adding other inducements. On Third Avenue a giant, glassy tower has slowly risen in the two years since he turned Stanford down—the $40 million research building to deepen Barrow's scientific presence among competing major neurological institutes.

With the drawn out wait over the Stanford offer ended, life at BNI settled back to its norm, never routine. Then suddenly, everyone thought last year that Spetzler's Phoenix years had come to an end. There was one job that never had been open, that even Spetzler never said he would refuse. In 1996, Charles Wilson announced his retirement as chairman of UCSF, Spetzler's residency alma mater. It was the one place he would never quite concede BNI could beat; the place built by the mentor he so admired.

When the dust cleared, Spetzler was offered the UCSF chairmanship. Again, Sonntag would be his deputy. In the months of considerations, one of Spetzler's top residents, Mike Lawton, was offered an attending staff job following his chief year. This was no easy decision, either way. For months they pondered, flew to San Francisco to talk, flew back. Many of the top members of BNI began checking housing prices in the Bay area, openly declaring that if Spetzler went, as surely he would, so would they. The prospect of a devastating drain on BNI's talent seemed certain.

Surprising even those who most wanted him to stay, Spetzler turned down the UCSF job.

The negotiations had at least one major, bright outcome. Lawton joined UCSF as an assistant professor.

How could Spetzler turn it down?

This was, he admits, far and away his toughest temptation ever. This was the one place that he knew would tempt him regardless of how good the offer was. And this was good. Sonntag was less interested in the move than Spetzler was. But in the end, he says, he had made too many commitments to his team at Barrow—notably the residents he had brought here with the promise that he would train them.

These are terrifically successful days, but not heady ones. In the new medical world, institutions that rest soon fall behind in the intensively competitive climate, no matter how "world-class" their reputations.

What has happened to costs of medical care at this high end in the past eight years is sometimes baffling. Salaries for those in training have remained entirely flat. Residents now make from $32,000 to $40,000 a year, as they did in the early nineties. Fellows, similarly, make just over $42,000 a year, and they are graduate neurosurgeons, frequently returning for a fellowship after practicing for a few years.

Among the attendings, the story is entirely different. National figures show that neurosurgeons average more than $430,000 a year in salary, double the figure as the decade opened. That might suggest that fees have similarly doubled, but they have not. Neurosurgeons earned $5,000 for performing a "standstill" procedure at the beginning of the decade. They now earn $6,200. Costs of other procedures similarly have crept up over the years but have not shown the great leaps of salaries. What accounts for the discrepancy? There is no ready answer, but a plausible one might be the ever-increasing numbers of neurological ailments and lesions that can be treated by neurosurgey; neurosurgeons may simply be busier than ever.

Perhaps the biggest change in the nineties is in hospital charges. Where once the rates for a particular surgery and recovery would not vary greatly from the national mean, now, as insurance companies arrive at allowable fees with a variety of different formulas, the charge for the same procedure and the same recovery period in the same hospital may vary between two patients by thousands of dollars—if they have different insurance companies. It is that competitive climate for patient dollars that forces hospitals around the country to keep up. Keeping up means many things to an internationally known center such as Barrow, but it most definitely includes keeping the "Yumas" of its patient population.

At the fringe of Barrow's coverage area, the BNI always has taken all neuro-surgery referrals from the regional medical center. But the city has no neuro-surgeon living there—a risk, considering it has a population of 80,000. Even more serious, that population doubles in winter with retirees, who have relatively high neurological problems. Twice before, neurosurgeons have hung out their shingles in Yuma, only to leave because of the lack of academic climate, or big city life, or prestige, or all of these.

Spetzler wants to persuade Yuma to remain in the BNI fold as its best option for assuring top neurological care. He wants to seek a neurosurgeon to take a position at Yuma that would include a partnership in BNI.

But he is not the only one wooing the medical staff. In southern Arizona, his friend Allan Hamilton, director of neurosurgery at the Arizona College of Medicine in Tucson, wants to provide coverage for Yuma as well. They are friends indeed, but in this they are competitors. And across the Colorado

River, California medical groups and hospitals as far away as San Diego are making pitches for Yuma.

The presentation on managing giant cranial aneurysms completed, Spetzler takes several questions. Then he makes his suggestions for neuro-surgical coverage by BNI and falls quiet. He listens for an hour as the mostly young physicians "openly and frankly" tell him what they love and hate about the idea. Can they afford an OR stocked, staffed and prioritized for neuro-surgery's demands when they now wait hours for OR space themselves? Alternatively, where would they get the wherewithal for new OR space? Will they still be able to send gravely ill and injured patients to Barrow, air-evacing them as they always have? Or will getting their own neurosurgeon ironically leave them less well-covered than before? Will an orthopedic surgeon be able to stay in business in competition with a neurosurgeon for all the spine cases? These days dollars coming into hospitals for specialty medicine are plummeting, sometimes in free fall on the charts. Whether they like this offer or not, can Yuma afford it?

NIGHT

Spetzler leaves on the last plane to Phoenix with the issue far from resolved, as he expected. But he tells Chief of Staff Mark Solovay over dinner that he is grateful for the openness of the conversation. At last the issues are out in the open and the discussions are truly under way.

It is black as pitch now on glass-smooth air returning to Phoenix, a rime of watermelon-colored light on the horizon all that is left of Wednesday. Tape recorder in hand, he holds one hand over his ear and shouts over the prop noise to get through his sheaf of paperwork. Landing is after 9 p.m. At 7:30 a.m. he will chair a BNI Board of Directors meeting. Then after a quick lunch it will be off to afternoon clinic, where he will meet patient Debra Lawson for the first time.

FRIDAY, JULY 25, 1997

At 7:00 a.m., Terry Steinberg, manager of the OR suite, is briefly alone, so the only sounds are hers, opening a drawer, writing with pen. Then another voice: "Are you always the first one in?"

"Only on Fridays, because Friday is Neurosurgery Clinical Conference. It'll last until almost 9:30."

"Look at that board!" A low whistle of disbelief. The Operating Room assignment board is crowded with chalked-in names, the neurosurgeon's in the second column after the OR number, then patient and procedure, then nursing and tech staff. Anesthesiologists usually spend the day in the same room as new cases come and go, so their names lie against a single OR number.

A cart comes down the hall punctuating the voices with its *skiek, skiek, skiek.* Background voices begin, a telephone rings. Morning rises with a clatter. On this day when Spetzler will attempt to clip "as dangerous an aneurysm" as he has ever seen, he is logged in for three other cases, and not an easy case among them. He moves from room to room on the board, as he will in reality, among rectangles already crowded with names of BNI surgeons and others with privileges here.

Names and surgeries march down the board, some annotated 'TF," to follow, meaning that they will begin after the previous case finishes, which in turn is dependent on the previous case, and so on down the day, far into the night and on into the weekend that once would see only emergency cases.

Carts carry supplies, doors unlock and open, slam shut, the heavy swinging outer doors whoosh loudly. More voices. A telephone. Two phones in discord and in the midst of one a voice calls over the loudspeaker: "...pick up line 1." A laughing voice, supply carts. The trauma bells and that soft, calm voice again. Now the din of the sterilizing room, roar of steam cleaners, motors, carts, clatter of fine high-grade steel.

Frances Rocha shouts over the of clash of instruments heading into the steam, over the whoosh of the cleaners. On request she displays the finest jewels in her charge: Spetzler's instruments. He has patented his own line of neurosurgical instruments and aneurysm clips, all made of pure titanium, a metal often used in supersonic aircraft because of its strength and lightness. They stand out among the tungsten because the metal glows with the prismatic iridescence of oil on water; to the touch they are light as a feather. Although weight was the most important consideration for the instruments, the major reason Spetzler picked titanium for the aneurysm clips is that it does not distort MRI images. Other metals throw shadows that can block vital information, or worse. Once a scanning procedure reportedly was fatal because the scanner's powerful concentrating magnet moved the clip. Manufactured and sold by a Swedish company, one Spetzler Aneurysm Clip costs $280. The instruments are being manufactured by a Missouri instrument company, which will sell the "Spetzler Tru-Micro Surgery Set" for a list price of $28,995. BNI gets the Spetzler instruments free.

In her twenty years at Barrow, Rocha has seen the operating room's standard supplies burgeon from two trays of instruments to seven. There are over one hundred different aneurysm clips in the neurosurgeon's armamentarium, bearing the names of their designers.

Out of the noise of the sterilizing room, voices and sounds are not the only collisions of morning. By 8:15, Steinberg already has her first scheduling emergency. A Spetzler patient who had a craniotomy for hemorrhage yesterday has begun to bleed again and must be brought back immediately. Spetzler has phoned with instructions to open up another OR, meaning that Steinberg must call in pool nurses to staff it and begin juggling the OR schedule. Spetzler is up to five procedures today, one an emergency. Steinberg says this is part of the new reality. While patients and neurosurgeons line up for available ORs, some remain closed by tight funding.

The door to OR 1 is propped open by a plain metal folding chair, on which stands a three-ring notebook labeled, "Debra Lawson, 2/12/59." At 9 a.m., the gurney bearing her wheels in, pushed and pulled by the blue-gowned nursing and anesthesia staff. Dressed in a pale blue hospital gown, she slides from gurney to table with help, trades a few jokes with Steve Cardon, her anesthesiologist. He talks to her all the while he is giving her the first of a series of anesthetics and barbiturates that will go on all day.

She closes her eyes as he talks, dozes, sleeps, and he slips on the face mask to begin inhalation anesthesia. Simply taken together the cocktail of numbing drugs given Lawson today would kill her. It is the difference between taking thousands of sounds and playing them in one deafening instant or stacking and stringing them into a symphony. These drugs will be dosed and timed with all the precision a decade's refinement has achieved, taking her down slowly, down farther, each moment a little closer to the bottom of the world. There she is to rest, but not cross over.

Though she is increasingly not here to appreciate it, she is now the center of a universe in extraordinary focus on her. By 9:25 a.m., eight nurses and technicians swarm around her still form in its swaddling hospital blankets. They affix wires, it seems, to every surface and appendage. Her eyes are taped shut. Large white patches on her ribs front and back are electrical terminals. They can deliver a charge to shock a wavering heart back to normal rhythm as the patient is re-warming and emerging from hypothermic arrest.

On her left middle finger, protruding from under the blue blanket, perches what appears to be a white clothespin, its interior glowing red around her finger. This is the business end of an ingenious measuring device. Just as children use flashlights to make hands and ears glow red, a beam of light from this clip passes through her finger. The spectrum of that light, which tells its composition, is read out on the other side. The major change as the light passes through her finger is that particular wavelengths of light are absorbed by the blood's oxygen, its signature. The difference between blood with more and with less oxygen is read by a computer as a light-spectrum change, converted into numbers, and posted on the anesthesiologist's monitor.

EKG leads for heart rate and rhythm are taped to both her arms and chest, and on her left arm there is a transducer to provide arterial blood pressure. A temperature lead probes her esophagus. Electrodes over the median nerve in her wrist send a steady beat of pulses up the spinal cord. The pulses are received by recording electrodes over the brain's somatosensory cortex— the sheet of neurons in the surface that takes in "touch" information. By monitoring those electrodes, the anesthesiologist can make sure that touch is being communicated to the brain.

An earpiece that might be from a Discman sends a steady stream of clicks inward to the brain stem, and those clicks had better evoke a response or there's major trouble. These "evoked potential readings," developed in the last decade by anesthesiologists including Peter Raudzens, are critical to skull-base neurosurgery. Passive EEG wires measure Debra's brain waves and will record their falling, dwindling to a calm, and the final moments when they will turn to a glassy frozen pond.

The last step is the Mayfield brace, a giant C-clamp with three prongs whose flat plates and sterile skull pins will fix her head absolutely still under any circumstance. The brace itself is affixed to the table. She is on her back, her face tilted 45 degrees to the left, toward the OR door. They will make the incision on the right, around the angular, skewed bone you can feel at your temple, and they will cut the top out of the right eye's bone mask, called the orbital ridge, to get to the bottom of the brain where it rests on its shelf behind the eyes, at the bridge of the nose. This approach will follow the third cranial nerve along the base of the brain to the X-crossing, the optic chiasm, that marks the circle of Willis, just as a pilot follows Interstate 8 to Yuma.

By 10:20, Spetzler has finished his emergency hemorrhage case and is going over films with Pam Smith. Carlos David, the neurovascular fellow, places a scalpel next to Lawson's right eye and draws a bright red arc incising her scalp.

The opening is under way, and it is one of the only times today that anyone will use that simple and inexpensive symbol of medicine, the surgical steel scalpel. From here on it will be the high tech tools of modern neurosurgery, the Midas Rex drill, electric cautery, computer-read wand, and most of the telemetry of mission control. This is the month of the Mars landing. The metaphor of space travel to a planetary brain had offered helpful, visual images less than ten years ago to describe the world emerging beneath the intraoperative microscope. Now those images have become reality. The instruments and precision-controls of space travel are here in the operating room. The mars lander fixed on stars to triangulate its position; NASA controllers used that position to determine a course, set by reference to those same stars. Here neurosurgeons fix on skull geography to triangulate structures in the brain, then use those structures to guide them down deeper within.

Together the cardiovascular and neurosurgical teams will guide one human brain to a landing, more gently than any spacecraft was ever guided to a remote cluster of rock in space. By Andy Warhol's prediction, everyone will get to be famous but only for fifteen minutes; this is the obverse prize. Debra Lawson will have more concentrated attention for one day than any monarch or pop star enjoys, but she won't know a bit of it. On the other hand, that's a far better gift when an aneurysm is about to kill you.

And the team huddled about the now-hidden form is only the visible emanation of what goes on here. Every wire and electric socket in the OR of today is on critical power—it will not fail in any emergency. The room is ventilated with a laminar air flow, meaning that it enters from ducts on one side and is drawn out on the far side. And that air is as clean as room air gets. Particles are removed down to one-half micron in size—a micron is a millionth of a meter—and the pollution tolerance allows for just one of these half-micron particles in every cubic centimeter of air.

Copper pipes supply the room with five lines of gas—oxygen, carbon dioxide, nitrogen, nitrous oxide, and medical air, which has been purified and filtered. The pipes must be sweated together in "super sterile" conditions by "super plumbers" so that pure and clean gases aren't contaminated in transit. The gases all come in pressurized to 50 pounds per square inch. A sixth pipe is a vacuum line. All the gases have been dehumidified except for the medical air, which must be breathable without drying out nasal and throat passages. High-pressure nitrogen runs the Midas Rex drill and other pneumatic tools, without causing corrosion.

Finally, the room itself is encased in hard-coated epoxy paint, and the floor is covered with welded sheet vinyl, impenetrable to blood stains or infectious agents.

Down in the basement of St. Joe's, the man who makes all these necessities into reality sits amid a neat array of the rolled up drawings and schematics that bear his name, Zoltan John Nagy, hospital architect. Most commercial building blueprints allow deviations from "true" lines by an eighth or even a quarter of an inch over distances. Nagy's typically make specifications within 1/256th of an inch. If vibrations occurred to even a tenth degree of those in a normal, solid building, the intraoperative scopes would offer only shimmering fields.

But it is Nagy's current project that offers his biggest headache and the best view into the future of neurosurgery. Plans are underway for a new neuro-surgery operating room, outside the BNI suite on the second floor. Currently, an intraoperative microscope with built-in "wand" pointer, video and still photo, and mouth controls costs from $300,000 up to half-a-million dollars. The new colossus costs $800,000. BNI pays far less, often nothing, because it is a developer of the tool. It will offer the neurosurgeon through-the-lens holog-raphy—three dimensional views of scans superimposed on a three-dimen-sional brain. And with it, Spetzler notes, comes a shifting of burdens for the surgeon. "You could easily get too much information in the operating field, which would interfere with your seeing the structures you're working on. So you have to decide in advance what you want to see where, and how much."

But the prospect, on the near horizon, is that while cutting on an opaque surface, the surgeon would know that two millimeters remained before a target tumor—or an exquisitely sensitive structure—would be reached.

Finally, the entire procedure can be projected from the OR into the BNI's Goldman Auditorium, where up to 200 onlookers in suitable glasses would be able to watch.

All this is still a means to bring greater safety to what remain massively invasive procedures. New technology hints at an eventual end to these.

The gamma knife quartered in the Research Building offers such a promise. Few pieces of equipment offer such contrasts in appearance and function between the archaic and the ultramodern. In concept, the $6 million machine works like a magnifying glass focusing the sun's rays to start a fire.

Gamma rays, which make up some of our dose of radiation from the sun and stars, can be fine tuned until they are powerful enough to destroy living tissue or weak enough to not even cause a tan. Lying in an enveloping sphere, the patient is the focus of gamma beams coming from the surrounding container from all directions. They rain down and all around the patient's head, though the beams are so weak they are harmless. The patient's head lies encased within a hemisphere of gleaming, brushed steel, thick enough to shield against the beams. However, the hemisphere is drilled with an array of 201 holes, so the whole looks like a very high-tech vegetable-draining colander. That means 201 separate gamma-ray beams stream into the patient's head. But the pattern and diameter of the holes cause the beams to focus on one single spot. Only at this point of focus are the rays powerful enough to destroy tissue. In minutes they can render a brain tumor lifeless while leaving surrounding tissue untouched.

There is no gamma knife for aneurysms. However, neurosurgeons at BNI and elsewhere have successfully blocked some aneurysm bulbs with only a small incision, and that not even in the head. They insert a super-fine catheter into an artery, usually in the groin, and carefully push the catheter up the artery into the brain. At the end of the catheter is a tiny strand of coiled metal, which looks like a very thin coil spring. When the filament reaches the aneurysm, it is rotated until this spring twists and coils against the inside walls of the bulb, entirely covering the bulb's walls on the inside. The aneurysm wall is now reinforced, and blood flows more normally through the open portion of the artery. The procedure holds a great deal of promise because of its safety, but it won't work on the giants like the one threatening Debra Lawson—at least not yet.

At 12:35 p.m., the massive, $800,000 microscope in its sterile plastic shroud was being rolled in, just as Spetzler returned from a quick lunch. "We just went under scope," David says.

"Open the Sylvian fissure completely," Spetzler says, a tall order and one that will bring the surgeons down to the basilar tip in the deep base of the brain. Picture the brain like a boxing glove, the rounded mitt being the cerebrum and the thumb the temporal lobe. The Sylvian or lateral fissure is the large valley between mitt and thumb. David will slowly work his way down through this gorge, separating the filmy arachnoid membrane, tugging back fine vessels, working his way along the third nerve toward the circle of Willis.

The high resolution, 3-D microscope once again delivers to the monitor the sense of walking into the brain itself, climbing downward into narrow rifts between the billowing white cerebral cortex webbed with bright red veins as David tugs and separates the filmy arachnoid membrane enveloping it. And once separated, a rift parts to reveal a breathtaking chasm lined with red and cobalt blue cables, the vascular blood structures whose treatment Spetzler and now David claim as their specialty. The relativity of depth and distance requires contrast for the mind to grasp what the eye sees. Fly at 30,000 feet on a clear day and you see only a flat, colored landscape at an indeterminate distance below. Then if you enter billowing trees of cumulus clouds and, through a sudden parting that reveals a lake of air, see the earth 30,000 feet below, it is a stunning vision.

And here, amid the white cortex that billows cloudlike, when a parting extends your view down twenty times the range you have been watching, you get a true sense of enormity. And that enormity belies the oddly mundane image of brain tissue surrounded by blue toweling that you can see directly just a few feet away, under David's gloved hands. The image on the monitor is, convincingly, the truer reality. Within that reality we follow the bright road of the oculomotor nerve from where we began just behind the right eye down to the optic chiasm, the X-crossing of right and left that marks the circle of Willis.

Suddenly, David parts the last membrane of the Sylvian fissure, and a chasm yawns profoundly enough to bring a touch of vertigo, laced down into its depth with thick and thicker cables, very dark blue, gun-metal ropes of blood vessels and billows of cerebral cortex. He uses scissors to pull small veins away. With the Sylvian fissure open all the way, we're looking down now into the circle of Willis itself, through a cavern with stalactites and stalagmites of cobalt blue, tiny arteries and veins.

All the way down to a glistening, rounded opalescent floor.

With a slight change in the position of the microscope, the basilar artery with its major feeder arteries come clear. That is no rounded floor gleaming angry and red at the basilar tip, though it's large enough, spans enough of this territory to be so. This "floor" is more like a lava dome, and at any moment it can blow up.

Such an aneurysm did earlier this summer. Just as Spetzler had begun seating a clip, the aneurysm broke. Blood filled every part of the operating field. Working quickly, he and his assistants managed to seal the rupture and get the bleeding controlled. The patient suffered relatively minor blood loss, although there is always a danger that blood irritation will bring on seizures later.

Heart surgeon Ravi Koopot has been at work for an hour. Lawson is now on bypass. Her heart long ago was stopped, but blood has been circulating all along propelled by the "heart-lung machine," the bypass pump.

It's time for the standstill, and now the chill in the room intrudes. The air temperature is already down to 60 degrees, and it's still dropping. Today it will only drop to 56, but it can be brought to near freezing. Three years ago architect Nagy designed and installed refrigeration to deliver laminar room air at 33 degrees Fahrenheit for the standstills. During trial runs, it began to snow in OR 1. It turned out that, even dehumidified, the air was too damp for such low temperature.

Back to the drawing board for Nagy, to further dehumidify the air. To cram in all the telemetry, pipes, electric cables, data wires and the usual ducts for heating, air conditioning and ventilation, above the ceiling of OR 1 Nagy had 11.5 inches of ceiling space to work with.

"The tricky part will be to dissect the dome of the aneurysm—the weakest part—to get at the clot," Spetzler says. "It must have bled before." By dissect he does not mean to cut the aneurysm open, but to separate it from the tendrils of perforators and membrane that surround it.

Spetzler must set the clip in the top of the V where the basilar tip arises from the vertebral arteries without disturbing the underlying blood vessels— the aneurysm is right at the joint. If you hold your fingers up in the V-victory sign, the fleshy area between the knuckles of your index and middle fingers is where the aneurysm swells outward toward you, the two fingers representing the vertebral arteries, with the aneurysm at the very place they combine to form the tip of the basilar artery. Imagine sliding a hairpin along the top of your hand to seal off the base of that knob that is half buried in the joint of the fingers. Now reduce the scale by thirty-five times and bury the whole model deep within tissue so delicate that instruments must never accidentally brush the wrong place, no matter how delicately. And every-where, of course, are the perforators, the tiny arteries that have become entangled with the huge, pressing balloon but which must not be included in the clip at the risk of stroke.

A week earlier Spetzler had put a clip on an aneurysm smaller and more clearly separated from an artery not so deep in the brain stem, and therefore not requiring a standstill. But as he tried to seat the clip, it repeatedly slid off the high-pressure balloon swelling within its pincers, each time risking a break that might be lethal. At each new slip, Spetzler murmured, "Don't break, don't break." Tense minutes went by as he maneuvered the clip before he finally seat-ed it. He then placed a second clip opposite the first, to ensure the seal. So the many risks of standstill were avoided in that surgery, but greater risks of hemorrhage were a clear and present danger.

In this light, at this angle, the angry red ball of Lawson's aneurysm has changed hue and is a giant pearl, occupying the whole screen in three dimensions.

Speaking to Cardon, Spetzler says, "Steve, how cold are we?" Cardon:

"Brain is at 30.8" centigrade, about 87 Fahrenheit. The room is now at 62 degrees, heading toward 55. Blasts of arctic air pour down from the ceiling; outside it is the usual 110 degrees of a Phoenix July afternoon. Cardon: "Brain is now 16.3." Down to 61 Fahrenheit.

Spetzler: "Go ahead and shut off and drain, please."

The blood-circulating, bypass pumps go quiet. It is 2:20 p.m., and the anesthesia of standstill is complete. Debra Lawson is chilled to the brain stem. No blood flows so the neurons are silent, beyond dormancy. Even the millions of cells that remain active during sleep are quiet now, and those millions that fire during unconsciousness, or during the heavy anesthesia of most neurosurgery when unconsciousness is profound. All are still. The EEG waves are flat as a glassy, frozen pond.

Each time you follow this journey down, you see things you didn't see before, within structures or wrapped around them or nested within, but it's never quite the same as what you saw before. It's all new and rises right before your eyes; that is the power of resolution. There is no end to it. The more you learn, the more you see, and what you see may contradict what you saw before, or may give it depth or refinement. That is one way to fit infinity into a six-inch hemisphere. Finally, somehow, a three-pound brain folded within that six-inch stone shell becomes the locus of one human consciousness.

Spetzler says, "See all those perforators down there?" Through the 3-D scope, the perforators look like roots coming through a drain pipe, fibers and tendrils everywhere, clustered around the very thick, ropy structures that are the arteries that Spetzler will have to deal with. The huge pearl is covered with these perforators, in front and, partly hidden, behind.

Now an abstract point becomes visible. As the blood drains after the bypass pump is shut off, the pearl collapses like a hot air balloon without heat, right there on the floor at the circle of Willis. There is no pressure in it, no movement, and Spetzler is now able, far easier than clipping the aneurysm in the usual way a week ago, to pull away the tiny perforators. He spends the better part of ten minutes doing nothing more, and explaining to the residents who are gathered around what each of the perforators is, or more often asking them to name where he is and what structures they're looking at.

But just as he's trying to seat the clip for the third time, he says, "Has she taken a breath?" Not literally of course, but it is the same effect: surprise. It's as though the respirator had been accidentally turned on, because he sees the aneurysm begin to refill, as it would if air had been forced into the lungs, causing pressure on the arteries and veins that would slowly spread out into the brain. Might the aneurysm somehow refill again? But no, the swelling subsides again.

It is exactly 2:30 when he reseats the clip. He asks how many minutes they have been under and the answer is, "You're at ten minutes"—not a long time. He stops trying to seat the clip, which is giving him trouble, and asks for "fenestrated clip number 6." He slips that one on with apparent ease. Then come his welcome words, "Start the pumps, please." Photographer Pam Smith has come in, and he says, "The clip is seated. Shoot." She clicks on the intra-operative camera. He moves the clip slightly, so that different views will show, and each time he does so says, "Shoot."

The pumps are started after eighteen minutes off; that is, she's actually been in hypothermic arrest for eighteen minutes, but then he asks for the pumps to be turned off once more so that he can make sure the clip is seated correctly and that in fact the aneurysm hasn't started to refill. It is still quiet. Is it quiet for good?

Spetzler says, "It looked like one of the perforators went under the clip, but it hadn't. But that's why you need to look, always look, on all sides of the aneurysm."

A nurse's voice: "Start re-warming?"

"Yes."

David: "I thought you had included a perforator there for a minute." And Spetzler goes back and shows him that it was not. But he says to David, "If you do this without hypothermic arrest, it's 100 percent certain, with this kind of aneurysm you will include perforators, there is no way to avoid it."

And David: "Everywhere else I've been, they'd have seen the perforators after getting down to the aneurysm, and they would have called the aneurysm unclippable."

Spetzler: "And so would I. Had I gotten down there, if it hadn't been for hypothermic arrest, I would have called this aneurysm inoperable."

David did his residency at top-flight Miami, where Roberto Heros and

Sidney Peerless are neurovascular stars. He says this fellowship concluding his training has been "spectacular." "The number, complexity, and degree of difficulty of aneurysms and other skull-base surgery here has been beyond anything I've ever seen before."

Lawson's return to life will be slow and steady, as carefully measured as the descent. She will remain on heart bypass for an hour or more, until her body has re-warmed above 86 degrees Fahrenheit; at that point Cardon can start her heart safely. But the watch will continue through several key stages of recovery. Finally, David will begin closing only when he is sure that the electrical activity of her brain is recovering; that's what this has all been about. David will stitch together the dura mater membrane, the toughest and outermost of the meninges, then screw the bone plate back in place, and stitch muscle together over it in two layers. He will pull up the forehead skin that had been tacked back, and stitch it back in place. By 6 p.m., Debra Lawson will be rolled out of OR 1, and the wait will begin.

Spetzler scrubbed out at 3:30, out to begin Friday rounds. He had done six cases today, including Debra Lawson's, two more than he'd anticipated. It was not until he and David stood with the residents gathered behind them, before the orange glow of the CT control terminal as the scans progressed before them that there was, really, closure. David sighed with relief. "It's never over until you can see that everything is okay," he said. The scans looked good. There was no bleeding. The aneurysm was history. The question now was one of recovery. At 6:15, Spetzler headed home.

RE-EMERGENCE

As evening falls in summer across much of the United States, you can watch fireflies begin to blink. A few at a time, hardly visible in the purple light, then growing in patterns until they form great sheets that flicker on and off to some orchestral conductor undetectable to humans. As morning comes, or on waking at any time, something like that happens in the brain. No light bulb blinks on. Rather, whole patterns of neurons fire, like fireflies in the brain's darkness. Soon—in seconds for most of us—whole sheets of "fireflies"

light in different patterns and "colors," some in different rhythms. Some
sheets lie parallel like higher and lower ocean currents. Others intersect like
a newspaper sheet on the wind, curling and diving then wrapping and
stretching out flat; but these are more like sheets of lights intersecting. It all
happens too fast to see, even if it could be filmed in the brain of a slow
waker. But if we could look into the brain of a patient emerging over days
out of the profound coma of standstill, there would be a world of time to
see it all happen. If we could only see neurons fire in their patterns, each as
a single flash, it would be the most dazzling light show in the cosmos.

But of course, it couldn't hold a candle to reality. Reality is what those
neurons' firing means to the person waking. The whole of the world grows
from a dimness to a wholeness of senses. Sounds, sights, smells; the feel of
things and their taste. Meaning. All the emotional coloring that humans bring
to these. All the thought that sometimes leads and sometimes runs behind.

Awake.

At his desk between two surgeries, Spetzler thrusts his hand out palm up,
fingers extended toward the ceiling. The fingers are perforator arteries.
"Imagine the aneurysm is a balloon in my hand, and it's swelling out, little by
little but with enormous pressure." Soon the balloon distends the perforator-
fingers, stretching them so taut that critical blood flow is reduced. Now the
brain stem begins to starve for oxygen. And onward the balloon swells "until
it actually envelopes the perforators, beginning to fuse its tissue with theirs."
Disaster is in the making, inexorably, in weeks or days.

"It is the most dangerous aneurysm I have ever seen," Spetzler says.
It is shutting down critical life functions for a 35-year-old surgeon. It was he
who approached Spetzler in Amsterdam and followed up with E-mail from
Katmandu, Nepal. Spetzler will attempt to separate out the perforators and
clip the aneurysm during a standstill on August 29. The patient's survival odds
are in the fifty-fifty range, Spetzler says; no better. It's safe enough to offer that
here in print. The outcome will be zero or one long before these words are
published. Spetzler is uncommonly blunt: "He'll be dead if he doesn't have this
done. And he may be dead if he does."

By squeezing the lifeblood of the brain stem, the aneurysm is shutting down the victim's ability to swallow, one of the most primitive functions. As the case of T.J. Mathias illustrated nine years before, the more primitive the function—heartbeat, breathing—the more essential it is to life itself.

And as in TJ's surgery, there is a significance to this operation beyond the outcome, though the outcome will always spell success or failure. Five years ago Spetzler would not have considered such an operation under any circumstances. His reason: He would not have been certain that a bad outcome resulted from the deadliness of the aneurysm rather than the standstill procedure, and that means the procedure could not have been done. *First, do no harm*—the prime commandment of the Hippocratic Oath. The physician cannot destroy the patient in an effort to save him.

The major change over the years, Spetzler says, is not in the numbers of standstills done, however large, but in the increasing difficulty of cases he is willing to tackle using the procedure. The BNI neurosurgeons have tuned the standstill until they can be confident that *it* is not causing morbidity and mortality. The outcome, in other words, is a product of the illness, not the doctor's efforts.

It is hard to imagine a case tougher than this. "I can get the aneurysm," he says. "I am very confident of that. I do not know what we can do to get the perforators functioning normally again, delivering a normal blood supply." On the other hand, he is equally confident that this is the patient's only chance.

DEBRA AND DANIEL LAWSON boarded a plane for Knoxville on August 20. She would become an outpatient at the Patricia Neal Rehabilitation Center there. Her soft drawl has returned, her speech is normal. She seems like someone getting over a serious bout with the flu, ailing but getting better. She is proud of Daniel's finishing high school in May, the first person among his grandmother's family to do so, and anxious for him to begin further schooling in the fall. She is returning to her family and step-family with some major mysteries remaining. Are their familial connections that might have predicted this aneurysm, or at least a propensity for it?

She has a family history of migraines, but migraines are not indicators of aneurysms. Dr. Kathern Plenge, director of neuro-rehabilitation for

St. Joseph's, says some people with familial arteriovenous malformations, AVMs, get migraines, but aneurysm sufferers do not. Lawson has a family history of cerebral hemorrhage, and those, of course, often are caused by rupturing aneurysms. But often not. Causes of death in the past were frequently left vague. Even now, deaths by cerebral hemorrhage rarely are traced to any precipitating cause.

But time has brought blessings to Lawson. Five years ago her aneurysm also would have been inoperable. Small changes at the operating end led to major differences in outcome.

Joe Zabramski, who still coordinates the research efforts, explains what the fine tuning has meant. Lesson one of the standstill: "Keep the time short and the temperature not too cold." They are playing off the advantages of the bloodless, visible operating field and the protectively low brain activity against the dangers of hypothermia and the risk that the brain cells' electrical dance will not come back all the way.

In practice, this means Spetzler now does as much work toward the aneurysm as possible before the heart bypass pump is turned off. Increasingly, all the OR preparations are made for the standstill but the radical procedure is not invoked until the last minute, when its necessity is certain, the time can be kept short, and the surgeon can still be confident of not destroying brain function as the deadly aneurysm is rendered harmless.

And now there is a new approach, modified at BNI, that accounts partly for the breathtaking depth seen during the operation that had not been there before. Formerly the surgeon lifted the brain from where it rests on the flat table of skull, gradually moving in toward the circle of Willis from below. That sometimes injured the brain, Spetzler says.

The new approach is more painstaking and slower but safer, bearing the tongue-twisting name of Orbitozygomatic. Parsed out it's not so hard to follow: the zygomatic bone arches over the temple; you can feel it there. The orbit is of the eye. The orbit and zygomatic are the bones Carlos David removed in opening. Then he spent hours parting the membrane between the temporal and frontal lobes, the thumb and mitt of the boxing glove. That's where the profound depth came, the plunge through a whole world, down through the Sylvian fissure between those major lobes. Following the third cranial nerve while trying to avoid irritating it, he and then Spetzler reached the brain stem.

So it will be again on the Friday before Labor Day. They will come right to the bone that thrusts up through the wide canal carrying the spinal cord. This bone, called the clivus, will be removed. The basilar artery, which lies against the clivus, now will be approached clearly and safely.

Better tactics will not be the only new weapons the team will bring to this next most-dangerous aneurysm. The telemetry NASA developed to carry Sojourner to Mars will guide their approach. The microscope will be the pointer that brings up scans of the patient's brain, and the scans will be melded to offer the operators the best of each technology. The bone structure delineated by the CT, the brain tissue revealed by the MRI, the metabolic activity shown in the PET scan all will be finely resolved and layered one on one. All will add to the growing confidence about what lurks at a hair's breadth behind the next shadow.

Each advance eventually reaches its limit, a point where, no matter how minute, the single thing critical to the living brain will not resolve further, where it will swell frustratingly into a great gray blob; and that will dictate a limit that no one, however skillful and confident, can breach. For now.

Then out of nowhere, if the past continues as predictor, tiny rivulets of discoveries, each seemingly insignificant, will unexpectedly merge in a rush, a river of achievement. *Voila.* The unbreakable barrier is breached. The gray blob is brought into a new, fine resolution and rendered as harmless as shadows in a spotlight.

That is the power of resolution: To never admit of a final *limit.* To never have to say *once and for all,* there is nothing more to be done— no matter how many times it has to be confessed. Resolution is limited, sometimes by the will and energy to see and the inventiveness of the seers, and it takes time to achieve in the best of worlds. New layers of the world that emerge at new resolutions open up only for those who will not let the gray remain so, but sometimes even the best of them is frustrated by the unyielding nature of reality.

The standstill is one marker telling where we stand in dealing with the brain by understanding some of its biology. But it is also a perfect place to start trekking into the mind, at the null place before sense or feeling. On our left is silence, straight ahead is nothing, all around the closest to quiet a human brain can be; all senses start here at zero. That the self can return from this origin whole and articulate, expressing its totality and parts, we have now seen over and over. It is not a miracle; it is a fact of science, brought about and witnessed by trained and measuring eyes. It tells a story of the hard nature of consciousness, the literal meaning of self, its geology and ecology. You either always knew the miracle or you still don't. What else is new?